Understanding
Diabetes

Professor Rudy Bilous

Published by Family Doctor Publications Limited
in association with the British Medical Association

With contributions from Andrea Miller, BSc, SRD, Lorna Hall, BSc and Debbie
Black, BSc, Senior Specialist Dietitians, South Tees Acute Hospitals Trust, and
Sharon Martin, Chief IV Chiropodist, Tees and North Yorkshire Community and
Mental Health Trust

Family Doctor Publications, PO Box 4664, Poole, Dorset BH15 1NN

ISBN-13: 978 1 903474 36 5
ISBN-10: 1 903474 36 1

19972009

Contents

About the author

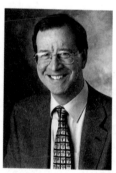

Professor Rudy W. Bilous is Professor of Clinical Medicine at Newcastle University and the South Tees Hospitals NHS Trust, researching into diabetic kidney disease and methods of achieving optimum blood glucose control. Professor Bilous was Chairman of the Professional Advisory Council Executive of Diabetes UK until September 2005.

Introduction

How widespread is diabetes?

If you have just found out that you have diabetes, this doesn't mean that you have become sick or turned into an invalid. Millions of people in this country have diabetes and most lead normal, active lives. Some have had the condition for over 50 years.

With advances in our understanding of the disease and improvements in treatment, the prospects for someone with diabetes are better than ever before. This book is meant to help you understand what diabetes is and how to control it.

Personal responsibility

Doctors nowadays encourage people with diabetes to take a lot of responsibility for their own health, paying careful attention to their diet and carrying out regular tests on their blood and urine in order to monitor their progress. We explain, step by step, how you can do this and how you can develop confidence that you really are in control of your diabetes.

The history of diabetes

Diabetes is one of the oldest known human diseases. Its full name – diabetes mellitus – comes from the Greek words for syphon and sugar, and describes the most obvious symptom of uncontrolled diabetes: the passing of large amounts of urine that is sweet because it contains sugar (glucose). There are descriptions of the symptoms by the ancient Persians, Indians and Egyptians, but a proper understanding of the condition has developed only over the last hundred years or so.

The discovery of insulin

In the later part of the nineteenth century, two German doctors worked out that the pancreas – a large gland behind the stomach – must be producing some substance that stopped the level of blood glucose rising.

In 1921 three Canadian scientists isolated the mystery substance, which they named insulin, from small groups of cells within the pancreas called the islets of Langerhans.

When insulin became available as a treatment for diabetes after 1922, it was seen as a medical miracle, transforming the future prospects of those with the condition, and saving the lives of many young people who would otherwise have died after a painful wasting illness.

Some 30 years later, it was found that one form of diabetes could be treated with tablets to lower levels of blood glucose. This new development led doctors to distinguish two forms of the condition.

The location of the pancreas

Insulin and glucagon are produced by specialised cells in the pancreas. This organ also secretes digestive enzymes into the gut; it is situated behind the stomach.

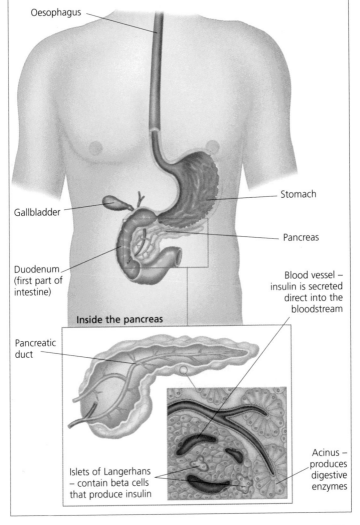

Oesophagus

Stomach

Gallbladder

Pancreas

Duodenum (first part of intestine)

Blood vessel – insulin is secreted direct into the bloodstream

Inside the pancreas

Pancreatic duct

Islets of Langerhans – contain beta cells that produce insulin

Acinus – produces digestive enzymes

Type 1 (insulin-dependent diabetes mellitus)

This starts most commonly in younger patients who have to have regular injections of insulin to remain well.

Type 2 (non-insulin-dependent diabetes mellitus)

Also called age-related or maturity-onset diabetes, this is more common in middle or later life and can be controlled by tablets or just diet.

What is diabetes?

Diabetes is a permanent change in your internal chemistry that results in you having too much glucose in your blood. The cause is a deficiency of the hormone insulin.

A hormone is a chemical messenger that is made in one part of the body (in this case the pancreas) and released into the bloodstream to have an effect on more distant parts.

There may be complete failure of insulin production as in type 1. In type 2, however, there is usually a combination of a partial failure of insulin production and a reduced body response to the hormone. This is called insulin resistance.

What goes wrong?

The glucose in your blood comes from the digestion of food and the chemical changes made to it by the liver. Some glucose is stored and some is used for energy. Insulin has a unique shape that plugs into special sockets or receptors on the surface of cells throughout the body. By plugging into these receptors, insulin makes cells extract glucose from the blood and also prevents them from breaking down proteins and fat.

It is the only hormone that can reduce blood glucose, and does this in several ways:

- By increasing the amount of glucose stored in the liver in the form of glycogen
- By preventing the liver from releasing too much glucose
- By encouraging cells elsewhere in the body to take up glucose
- By preventing cells elsewhere in the body from breaking down protein and fat.

Other mechanisms in the body work together with insulin to help maintain the correct level of blood glucose. Insulin is the only means that the body has of actually lowering blood glucose levels, however, so, when the insulin supply fails, the whole system goes out of balance. After a meal, there is no brake on the glucose absorbed from what you've eaten, and the level in your blood goes on rising. When the concentration rises above a certain level, the glucose starts to spill out of the bloodstream into the urine. Infections such as cystitis and thrush (candida infection) can develop more easily when the urine is sweet because the germs responsible can grow more rapidly.

Passing more urine

Another consequence of rising blood glucose is a tendency to pass more urine. This is because the extra glucose in the blood is filtered out by the kidneys, which try to dispose of it by excreting more salt and water. This excess urine production is called polyuria and is often the earliest sign of diabetes.

The effect of insulin in a healthy person

After a meal blood glucose levels rise. In a healthy person, the pancreas responds to this by producing more insulin, which has the following effects in the body.

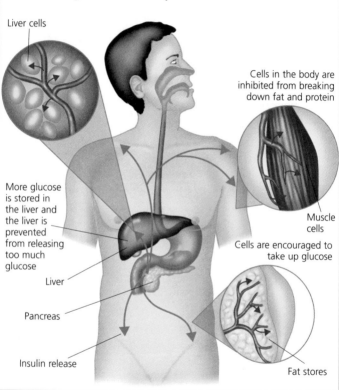

Liver cells

Cells in the body are inhibited from breaking down fat and protein

More glucose is stored in the liver and the liver is prevented from releasing too much glucose

Liver

Pancreas

Insulin release

Muscle cells

Cells are encouraged to take up glucose

Fat stores

If nothing is done to halt this process, the person will quickly become dehydrated and thirsty. As previously mentioned, as well as regulating blood glucose, insulin acts to prevent weight loss and help build up body tissue – so a person whose supply has failed or isn't working properly will inevitably lose some weight.

Symptoms of diabetes

The severity of the symptoms and the rate at which they develop may differ depending on which type of diabetes you have. Symptoms caused by type 1 and type 2 diabetes:

- Thirst

- Dehydration

- Passing large quantities of urine

- Urinary tract infection (such as cystitis) or thrush

- Weight loss

- Tiredness and lethargy

- Blurred vision resulting from dehydration of the lens in the eye.

Ketoacidotic coma

Type 1

As the person isn't producing any insulin at all, the symptoms can come on very rapidly because internal blood glucose control is lost.

Insulin has a very important role in maintaining stability in the body by preventing breakdown of proteins (found in muscle) and fats. When insulin fails, the byproducts of the breakdown of fat and muscle build up in the blood and lead to the production of substances called ketones. If nothing is done to stop this, the level will rise, until eventually it causes the person to go into what's called a ketoacidotic coma.

This is much less common these days because diabetes is usually diagnosed long before coma develops. However, when it occurs patients need urgent hospital treatment with insulin and fluids into a vein. This is not the same thing as a coma induced by low blood sugar (or hypoglycaemia) – see page 76.

Type 2

As the supply of insulin is reduced or is not quite as effective as normal, the blood glucose level rises more slowly. There is less protein and fat breakdown so ketones are produced in much smaller quantities, and the risk of a ketoacidotic coma is lower.

Who gets diabetes?

Almost four per cent of people in this country have diabetes, although as many as half of them may not realise it. This number is steadily increasing. The vast majority have type 2, and more women than men are affected, probably because diabetes is more common later in life and women tend to live longer. As the age of the population as a whole is rising, type 2 diabetes is likely to become even more common over the coming years.

In addition, the incidence of diabetes is increasing worldwide and is estimated to result in a near doubling of the population with type 2 diabetes by 2025. Moreover, children in the UK seem to be developing type 1 diabetes at an earlier age, and there are increasing numbers of patients developing type 2 diabetes in early adulthood.

What causes diabetes?

There are many reasons why insulin secretions may be reduced and an individual could be affected by more than one cause.

Estimated diagnosed diabetes by type and country for the UK

Nation	Type 1	Type 2	Total number in 2005
England	211,000	1,555,000	1,766,000
Scotland	20,000	147,000	167,000
Wales	13,000	104,000	117,000
Northern Ireland	7,000	46,000	53,000
Total UK	**251,000**	**1,852,000**	**2,103,000**

Genetic

Researchers studying identical twins and the family trees of patients with diabetes have found that heredity is an important factor in both kinds of diabetes. With type 1 diabetes, there is about a 50 per cent chance of the second twin developing the condition if the first one has it, and a 5 per cent chance of the child of an affected parent developing it.

With type 2 diabetes, it is virtually certain that, if one of a pair of identical twins develops it, the other will do so as well.

It is difficult to predict precisely who will inherit the condition. A small number of families have a much stronger tendency to develop diabetes and scientists have identified several genes that seem to be involved. In these circumstances, it may be possible to test family members and determine their risk of developing the condition. For the most part, however, it is difficult to identify the genes involved and this makes it different from some other conditions such as cystic fibrosis, where a single gene is operating.

So even if a close member of your family has diabetes, there is no certainty that you will develop it yourself. Some people who inherit a tendency to diabetes never actually get it, so there are obviously other factors at work here.

Infection

It has been known for some time that type 1 diabetes in children and young people is more likely to come on at certain times of the year when there are a lot of coughs and colds about.

Some viruses, such as the mumps virus and Coxsackie virus, are known to have the potential to damage the pancreas, bringing on diabetes. As far as individual patients are concerned, however, it is very rare that doctors can link the onset of their diabetes with a specific bout of infection. A possible explanation for this is that the infection may have begun a process that comes to light only many years later.

Environment

People who develop type 2 diabetes are often overweight and eat an unbalanced diet. It's interesting to note that people who move from a country with a low risk of diabetes to one where there's a higher risk have the same chance of developing diabetes as the locals in their new country.

There is a close link between body weight and the development of type 2 diabetes. Recent surveys have shown a dramatic increase in obesity in the UK, especially in young people, and this is partly responsible for the increasing incidence of diabetes.

A good example of this is shown by the Pacific islanders of Nauru who became very wealthy when phosphates were discovered on their island. As a consequence, their diets changed dramatically; they put on a lot of weight and they became much more prone to developing diabetes.

All this points to important connections of diet, environment and diabetes. However, there is no precise link between developing diabetes and the individual consumption of sugar and sweets.

Secondary diabetes

There are a small number of people who develop diabetes as a result of other disease of the pancreas. For example, pancreatitis (or inflammation of the pancreas) can bring on the condition by destroying large parts of the gland. Some people with hormonal diseases, such as Cushing's syndrome (the body makes too much steroid hormone) or acromegaly (the body makes too much growth hormone), may also have diabetes as a side effect of their main illness.

It can also be a result of damage to the pancreas caused by chronic over-indulgence in alcohol. Some long-term treatments such as steroids and beta-blocker tablets are also associated with an increased rate of development of diabetes.

Stress

Although many people relate the onset of their diabetes to a stressful event such as an accident or other illness, it is difficult to prove a direct link between stress and diabetes. The explanation may lie in the fact that people see their doctors because of some stressful event, and their diabetes is diagnosed opportunistically at the same time.

KEY POINTS

- Diabetes arises when either an individual cannot make enough insulin or the insulin that an individual does make is ineffective at controlling blood glucose levels

- Insulin is a hormone (chemical messenger) that is critical for maintaining healthy life

- Symptoms of diabetes are weight loss, passing more urine, thirst and feeling run down

- There are several causes including genetic (inherited) predisposition, infections, obesity, environmental factors and possibly stress, and any or all of these may be important in each individual case

- Being overweight greatly increases your chances of developing type 2 diabetes

Making a diagnosis

Discovering that you have diabetes
People find out they have the condition in different ways. With type 2, the first port of call is usually your GP, either because you have some or all of the symptoms listed on page 7, or because you are having a general check-up.

Some people are advised to see their doctor by their optician (or optometrist). This is because an eye examination will pick up the early signs of a condition called diabetic retinopathy – changes in the blood vessels of the eye that can develop as a complication of diabetes (see page 110).

Tests for diabetes
If your symptoms suggest to your doctor that you may have diabetes, he or she will want to do a blood test to measure your glucose level, and will also ask for a urine sample to be tested. The samples may have to be sent off to the lab for analysis, although most GPs today have blood glucose meters in the surgery, and can give you the result on the spot. Some pharmacies

Optometrist

Diabetes is often diagnosed by chance as the result of a visit to the optician (or optometrist), because an eye examination will detect diabetic retinopathy.

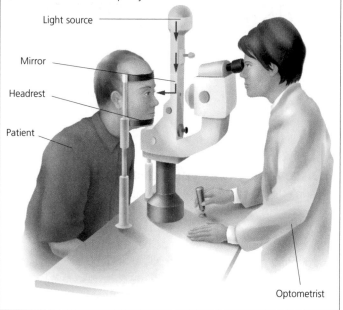

Light source

Mirror

Headrest

Patient

Optometrist

are also offering blood tests for people who are worried that they may have diabetes.

The structure of diabetes care

Above-average readings from either or both of these tests will probably be sufficient for your doctor to confirm that you have diabetes and, if it's type 2, it's likely that you will be cared for by your GP rather than having to see a hospital doctor.

Many GP practices run regular diabetes clinics but, if yours doesn't or you feel that you need more support, you can ask to be referred to a hospital diabetes clinic.

Fingerprick blood test

A simple fingerprick blood test will determine your blood glucose level.

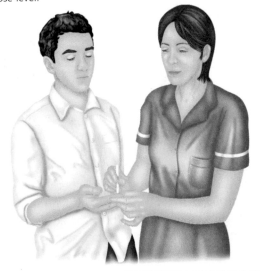

As mentioned above, type 1 diabetes can often come on quite suddenly, and this may mean the person being admitted to hospital while the diagnosis is made and the condition stabilised.

People with this form of diabetes will often continue to be under the care of the specialist team at a hospital. Nowadays, many patients with type 1 and type 2 diabetes have shared care between the hospital and the GP.

Although, for most people, the diagnosis is straightforward and quite clear cut, a few may need an extra test because their blood glucose level is borderline. In this case, you may be asked to have an oral glucose tolerance test. After an overnight fast, your blood glucose level will be measured on arrival at

Oral glucose tolerance test

If your blood tests show that your blood glucose level is borderline you may need an oral glucose tolerance test. There are three possible outcomes, depending on the results of your test:

1. Your blood glucose may be within the normal range, so you don't have diabetes.

2. Your level may be higher than average, although not high enough to mean that you have diabetes. This condition is called impaired glucose tolerance (IGT) and your medical advisers will want to keep an eye on you because there is a possibility of developing diabetes in the future. In the meantime you will be given advice on diet, although you don't have diabetes and don't need any other specific treatment.

3. Your blood glucose level may be sufficiently raised to indicate that you do have diabetes. If so, you will need to see your doctor to discuss what treatment you need.

the clinic; then you'll be given a drink containing a measured amount of glucose. Your blood will be re-tested at two hours to see how your body is dealing with the glucose that you've absorbed. You may also be asked to pass a urine sample at the start and end.

Testing urine

You may be asked by your doctor to provide a urine sample. This will be tested for glucose levels.

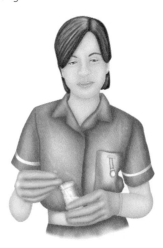

KEY POINTS

■ Diabetes is usually diagnosed from a simple urine or blood test in patients who have symptoms (see page 7)

■ A small number of patients need to have a more formal test called an oral glucose tolerance test

■ Early diagnosis is very important and patients with symptoms are recommended to attend their GP's surgery or local pharmacy for a test

Treatment: diet

Coping with diabetes

Diabetes can be tackled in three main ways.

Diet

A diabetic diet actually means following a healthy eating plan rather than a difficult or restrictive programme. This applies to everyone with diabetes, regardless of which type they have, and may be enough by itself to control type 2 in some people.

However, if you have type 1 diabetes, you will need to learn about balancing your intake of food with your insulin injections in order to achieve the best possible control of your blood glucose levels.

Tablets

These are used to control type 2 and there are different types. For more about this kind of treatment, see page 44.

Insulin

Everyone with type 1 diabetes will have to take insulin by injection, but only a minority of those with type 2 diabetes will be treated this way. More about insulin on page 49.

Your healthy eating plan

The sort of diet that you should follow when you have diabetes definitely does not mean a future of self-denial on the food front. What it does mean is eating more of the foods that are good for you, and cutting right down on those that are not so good. Actually it's the kind of eating that experts recommend for everyone, whether or not they have diabetes.

The difference that it can make to your overall health and well-being is even more worthwhile when you do have diabetes, however, because without it your medication will not be nearly as effective.

A balanced diet

It is important to have a good mix of foods so eat a wide range of different nutrients; also try to cut back on those that are high in fat and sugar. Once you get used to the basics, however, it's mostly quite simple, as you will see from our guidelines on the next few pages.

Eat regular meals

You should find it easier to keep your blood glucose levels under control if you eat at regular mealtimes. This may also be beneficial to aid weight loss. Aim to have three meals per day or eat approximately every four hours, that is breakfast, lunch and evening meal (see 'Healthy eating menu', page 20).

Some people may need to have a small snack, for example cereal or toast or snacks between meals, but this should be discussed with your diabetes team.

Healthy eating menu

A well-balanced diet helps control your diabetes and
ensures that your medication works effectively. This
chart will give you some ideas for the foods that you
should include in your meals.

Breakfast

- Skimmed or semi-skimmed milk
- Artificial sweetener instead of sugar
- High-fibre cereal, e.g. porridge, Branflakes,
  Weetabix, Shredded Wheat
- Wholemeal or wholegrain bread
- Poly- or monounsaturated or low-fat spreads
- Low-sugar jam or marmalade
- Fruit

Main meal

- Include some starchy food – bread, potatoes,
  pasta, rice or chapatti, for example
- At least two portions of vegetables, and try to
  include peas and beans as often as possible
- Small portions of lean meat or fish. Cut off fat,
  and avoid frying
- Fresh or tinned fruit (in natural, unsweetened
  juices), plus unsweetened/sugar-free jelly or
  custard

Snack meals

- Bread, pasta, chapatti or jacket potatoes – go for
  low-fat fillings such as lean meat, baked beans,
  low-fat cheese or tinned fish (not in oil)
- Fresh or tinned fruit in natural juice

Eating between meals

Snacks/Supper
- Avoid eating too many of these if you're trying to lose weight, and stick to fruit instead
- Sandwiches or toast with low-fat fillings
- Bowl of cereal or porridge
- Low-fat crisps
- Plain biscuits
- Toasted crumpets and muffins

The different food types
Carbohydrates

There are different types of carbohydrate, which are broken down by the body at different rates to produce glucose (sugar). In simple terms a carbohydrate can raise blood glucose levels dramatically (quick release), moderately or a little bit (slow release). Foods that have only a slow release have a small effect on blood glucose, whereas those with a quick release cause a rapid and massive rise in blood glucose level.

Try to have some slower-release carbohydrates at each meal, because they are a good source of energy and help to fill you up. They can also keep your blood glucose levels stable. Slow-release carbohydrates can be found in bread, pasta, rice, chapattis, breakfast cereals, potatoes, and so on.

Sugary foods are digested quickly and are rapidly absorbed into your bloodstream and increase your blood glucose levels, for example sugar, sweet fizzy drinks, sweets and chocolate, cakes and biscuits. There is no harm in having these foods occasionally but try to

How much to eat of each food type

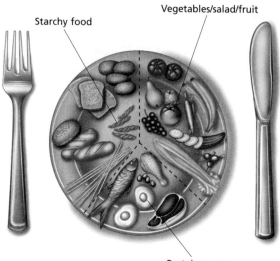

Starchy food

Vegetables/salad/fruit

Protein source

At each meal your food contribution needs to be in the above illustrated proportions.

Two-fifths of your plate should be covered with starchy food preferably of high-fibre variety (e.g. wholemeal bread, potatoes, pasta and rice).

Two-fifths of your plate should be covered with vegetables/salad or fruit.

The remaining one-fifth of your plate should be a protein source, e.g. meat, fish, eggs, pulses or cheese.

By ensuring that these proportions of nutrient sources are achieved and maintained, your blood glucose should stay within desirable ranges.

Slow-release carbohydrates

Bread, pasta, rice, chapattis, breakfast cereals, potatoes and fruit.

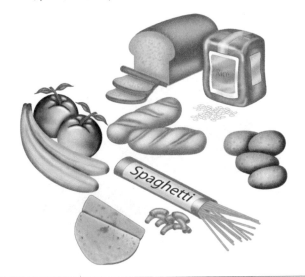

take sugar-free or low-sugar alternatives. Use diet or no-added-sugar drinks, have plain biscuits and cakes occasionally, and limit portion size.

The best time to have something sweet is with or after a main meal because the sugar is more slowly absorbed with other food types.

Modify your favourite recipes to use less sugar, for example cakes. Sugary foods are high in calories so it is best to limit these foods if you are concerned about your weight.

Carbohydrate counting

As carbohydrate is the main immediate source of glucose from the diet, there is a school of thought that suggests that people with diabetes should try to calculate

Sugary carbohydrates

Avoid or limit sugary carbohydrates as they will cause a sudden rise in blood glucose level.

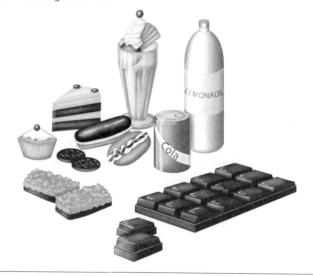

how much there is in each meal and adjust the insulin dose accordingly. Thus, a meal with more carbohydrate would need a larger dose of insulin and vice versa.

This system is called carbohydrate counting and is particularly useful for patients using multiple insulin injections (see page 53) or an infusion pump (page 61). The convention is to have 1 unit of insulin for every 7 to 20 grams of carbohydrate, depending on age and body size.

This method is similar to the old system of carbohydrate exchanges but does not involve a daily limit on the amount in the diet. It is simply a method of trying to match insulin dose to meal size.

The table opposite shows examples of the amounts of some common foods that are equivalent to

Portions of foods equivalent to 15 grams of carbohydrate

Bread and cereals
One slice wholemeal
Six dry crackers
One muffin/hot dog roll/hamburger bun
25 grams (1 oz) unsweetened cereal

Vegetables
50 g (2 oz) cooked Brussels sprouts, carrots, leeks, cabbage, cauliflower
Mashed potato – 100 g
Chips – 50 g (equivalent to 16–25)
Half a medium-sized baked potato
Cooked rice 50 g (2 oz)
Pasta – 70 g (2.5 oz)
Double quantity for raw portions

Fruit
One apple (150 g)
One large orange
One small banana
Half a grapefruit
Two kiwi fruit

Drink
Fruit juice 150 ml (3 oz)
Beer 1 pint
Milk half a pint (any type)

15 grams of carbohydrate. This system has been tested in a large research study sponsored by Diabetes UK – the Dose Adjustment For Normal Eating (DAFNE) Project.

By teaching type 1 patients how to adjust insulin to the carbohydrate content of an unrestricted diet, blood glucose levels were much better controlled at the end of one year than in a group of patients in whom this training had been delayed. It is planned to extend this programme across the UK.

For type 2 patients, a programme called DESMOND (Diabetes Education and Self-Management for Ongoing and Newly Diagnosed) has shown promising results. More information can be obtained from Diabetes UK (see page 147).

Fat

A diet rich in fat can lead to weight gain, raise blood cholesterol and contribute to heart disease. It can also make the body less responsive to insulin. There are two main types: saturated and unsaturated fat.

Saturated (animal) fat

This is found in butter, lard, fatty meats, pastries, and so on. This type of fat can increase your cholesterol level (see 'If it gets complicated', page 107). It is therefore important to reduce the intake of these types of foods. Instead try to increase the amount of fruit and vegetables, pulses such as lentils and beans, oily fish and oats.

Unsaturated fats

These are slightly better for you than saturated fats and come in two forms:

1   Polyunsaturated fats are found in sunflower oil,

pure vegetable oil, corn oil and sunflower margarines. They have little effect on cholesterol levels.

2 Monounsaturated fats are found in olive oil and olive oil-based margarines, rapeseed and safflower oil, and most nuts. This type of fat is thought to be most beneficial because it may reduce blood levels of your 'bad' cholesterol (low-density lipoprotein or LDL for short) and increase your 'good' cholesterol (high-density lipoprotein or HDL for short). This type of fat should be used instead of saturated or polyunsaturated, whenever possible.

Trans-fatty acids are formed when fats undergo a chemical process to make them hard, termed

Fat in foods

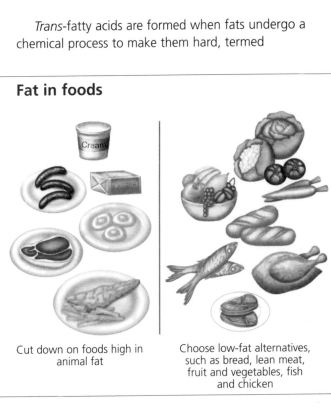

Cut down on foods high in animal fat

Choose low-fat alternatives, such as bread, lean meat, fruit and vegetables, fish and chicken

'hydrogenation'. *Trans*-fat raises LDL-cholesterol and lowers HDL-cholesterol levels, and so can increase the risk of heart disease. It is therefore important to limit the amount of foods containing them.

They are found mainly in hard margarine, crackers, biscuits, cakes, fried foods, pastries, baked goods and other processed foods made with or fried in partially hydrogenated oils. They may also be found in small amounts in various meat and dairy products.

Remember that all fats are high in calories and may lead to weight gain if taken in excess.

Oily fish

Oily fish such as mackerel, herring, kippers, salmon, trout, sardines and pilchards contain beneficial oils known as omega-3 (or ω-3) oils. Research has shown that these oils help to reduce the stickiness of the blood and lower cholesterol levels.

They may also protect against heart disease by helping the heart beat more regularly and protecting blood vessels. They are also thought to be beneficial in reducing inflammation and can help reduce arthritis symptoms.

Despite the recent research suggesting only a modest benefit, dietary experts recommend trying to have oily fish once or twice a week. Buy them fresh, tinned in brine (tinned tuna does not count because the omega-3 oil is destroyed during processing) or in tomato sauce, but avoid fish in any type of oil.

There are omega-3 supplement capsules available, which contain beneficial fish oils. However, there is not enough evidence to support their use in people with diabetes at the moment and they are expensive. It is best to obtain oils from fish themselves rather than from supplements.

If you do not like fish, then try the following instead: green leafy vegetables, nuts and seeds or omega 3-enriched foods, for example Columbus eggs.

Fibre

Fibre (also called roughage) can be either soluble (dissolves in water and slows absorption of food) or insoluble (cannot be digested and helps to prevent constipation). Insoluble fibre is also useful when you are trying to lose weight because it makes you feel full up.

Fibre

Consume plenty of fruit as well as vegetables and wholemeal cereals to keep the bowels working properly.

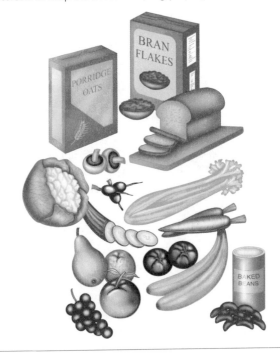

What is a portion?

Nutrition professionals often advise the inclusion of a certain number of portions of food types in the diet. This chart shows examples of the portion sizes of particular foods.

Food	Quantity to make a portion
Fruit and vegetables	
Melon, pineapple, half a grapefruit	One slice of large fruit
Banana, apple, orange	One medium fruit
Plums, tangerines	Two small fruit
Grapes, cherries, berries	One handful
Dried fruit	Half to one tablespoon
Pure unsweetened fruit juice	One small glass
Any vegetable	Two tablespoons
Salad	One small bowl
Milk and dairy food	
Milk (preferably semi-skimmed or, better still, skimmed)	One medium glass, 200 ml (a third of a pint)
Yoghurt, plain or flavoured, low fat and low sugar	1 small pot, 150 grams (5½ oz)
Cheese – preferably low fat	One matchbox size, 25 grams (e. Brie, Camembert, Edam, reduced fat Cheddar). The mini-portion si cheeses are handy
Cream cheese – light	The size of two small matchboxes, 80 grams (3 oz)

What is a portion? (contd)

Food	Quantity to make a portion
Milk and dairy food (contd)	
Cottage cheese	One small pot, 100 grams (3½ oz)
Fromage frais – light	One small pot, 150 grams (5½ oz)
Meat, fish and alternatives	
Sausages	Two grilled
Lean meat like beef, pork, ham, lamb, chicken (without skin) or oily fish	50–100 grams (2–3½ oz)
Cooked cold meat	Two slices
Fish – white or tuna in brine	100–150 grams (3½–5½ oz)
Fish fingers	Three
Eggs	Two
Baked beans in tomato sauce (low sugar and salt if possible)	200 grams or five tablespoons
Lentils	Four tablespoons cooked
Beans, e.g. red kidney beans, butter beans, chick peas	Four tablespoons cooked
Nuts	Two tablespoons
Peanut butter	Two tablespoons

Advice to help you get the most out of your food

Handy tips

- Have fruit or vegetables with every meal and have as snacks between meals

- Add extra vegetables to casseroles, curries, soups

- Add fruit to breakfast cereals

Cooking tips

- Cook vegetables for a short time in a little water to avoid destroying the vitamins and minerals

- Try microwaving, steaming or stir frying vegetables in a small amount of oil

Increasing the fibre content of your diet doesn't mean having brown rice and bran with everything, but you should aim to consume around 30 grams of fibre a day. It is essential to keep your intestine working well, and some food types such as soluble fibre can help with both good blood glucose control and keeping your blood cholesterol levels down.

Soluble fibre foods

Foods such as baked beans, mushy peas, lentil soup and dhal, plus oat-based dishes such as porridge and other cereals and oat cakes, are high in soluble fibre.

Insoluble fibre foods

Food such as high-fibre cereals, wholemeal or granary bread, unpeeled vegetables and fruit, plus wholemeal versions of pasta, flour and rice, have mainly insoluble fibre.

The importance of water

If you increase the fibre content of your diet it is important to increase fluid. Aim to drink eight to ten glasses of fluid per day – for example, squash with no added sugar, water, tea – because this helps to soften your motions and prevents constipation.

Fruit and vegetables

These are important, because they are low in fat and calories and provide plenty of vitamins, minerals and fibre. All fruit contains a small amount of natural sugar. It is therefore important that you spread your fruit intake over the day in order to minimise the amount of sugar that you take in at any one time.

It is recommended that you aim for five portions per day. This may help to protect against heart disease and decrease cholesterol levels. Fresh, frozen and tinned fruit in natural juice are all suitable. Potatoes are not usually counted as a vegetable portion but they are of course an important source of carbohydrate. If you are eating a well-balanced diet, you really should not need to take any extra vitamin or mineral supplements.

Protein

Protein is an important part of your diet because it is required for repair of tissue and muscle and is needed to fuel normal growth in children. You need only a relatively small amount – look up the value in the table on page 34.

Good sources of protein include eggs, fish, meat and dairy produce. Some of these foods can be high in fat, so it is important to use low-fat or diet versions when you are able to.

Protein requirements

The recommended amount of protein in your daily diet is determined primarily by your age and sex. The figures set out in the table below are the estimated average requirements (EARs).

Children		Men		Women	
Age (years)	Grams per day	Age (years)	Grams per day	Age (years)	Grams per day
< 1	11.0 g	11–14	33.8 g	11–14	33.1 g
1–3	11.7 g	15–18	46.1 g	15–18	37.1 g
4–6	14.8 g	19–50	44.4 g	19–50	36.0 g
7–10	22.8 g	50+	42.6 g	50+	37.2 g

The World Health Organization (WHO) does not give figures for 0–3 months, so no EAR can be derived. To save confusion, all babies aged under 1 year have been put together.

Examples of foods providing approximately six grams of protein

Milk (whole)	200 ml
Egg	1 medium/size 3
Baked beans	6 tablespoons
Red meat	20 grams
Chicken	25 grams
Cheese	25 grams
Pasta	50 grams

Salt

Too much salt can increase your blood pressure (known as hypertension). You should not eat more than six grams (one heaped teaspoon) of salt per day. If you suffer from hypertension then you should eat less than three grams of salt per day (half a teaspoon). To calculate how much salt is in a product, multiply the sodium level (often found on the label of tins or packets) by 2.5.

Try to taste your food first. You may not need to add salt; instead use herbs, spices, lemon juice, pepper, garlic, and so on. Do not add salt in cooking or at the table. There is a lot of salt hidden in processed food such as tinned or ready-made meals, cured meats, pizzas, and so on, so try to eat less of these. Cut down on salty snacks such as crisps and salted/toasted nuts.

Special diets

High-protein/low-carbohydrate diets are marketed by some as being particularly good for individuals who wish to lose weight. There is some scientific basis for these claims, but, if you are on any form of tablet or insulin treatment, you should get expert advice from your diabetes team before starting such a diet. A dramatic reduction in carbohydrate intake might result in hypoglycaemia (see page 76).

High-protein diets may have a long-term damaging effect on the kidneys, particularly in patients with proteinuria and early kidney failure (see page 113). Until the long-term safety of these diets is confirmed a balanced intake of a mixture of proteins, carbohydrates and fats, as outlined above, is still the safest choice.

Diabetic foods

It is better to avoid those foods such as diabetic chocolate, sweets and jam because they offer no benefits to people with diabetes. They can cause diarrhoea if eaten in large quantities because they contain a sweetener called sorbitol, which is not absorbed. They can also be high in fat and are expensive.

Controlling your weight

Type 2 diabetes is often associated with being overweight and obesity can make it more difficult to control blood glucose. If you are overweight (see chart opposite) then losing some weight will be beneficial to your health. Even losing just 10 per cent of your body weight can make huge improvements to your health by improving your diabetes control, blood pressure and cholesterol levels.

Remember that you will lose weight only if you eat less food than your body needs to fuel its daily activities. You may find it easier to introduce changes gradually rather than all at once. Your family may like to be involved and change their diet in order to eat more healthily. Our healthy eating menu (see page 20) shows how you might do this; substitute the foods listed for your usual ones.

Try these tips to lose weight

- Cut down on fried and fatty foods (see page 26)
- Eat smaller portions
- Cut out snacks such as crisps and biscuits; try fruit instead
- Eat regular meals
- Take more exercise

What should you weigh?

- The body mass index (BMI) is a useful measure of healthy weight
- Find out your height in metres and weight in kilograms
- Calculate your BMI like this:

$$BMI = \frac{\text{Your weight (kg)}}{[\text{Your height (metres)} \times \text{Your height (metres)}]}$$

$$e.g. \ 24.8 = \frac{70}{[1.68 \times 1.68]}$$

- You are recommended to try to maintain a BMI in the range 18.5–24.9
- The chart below is an easier way of estimating your BMI. Read off your height and your weight. The point where the lines cross in the chart indicates your BMI

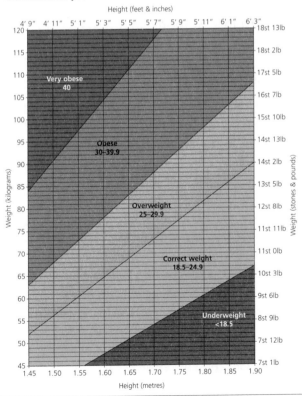

If you would like to discuss any of these points or would like more information, ask your doctor to refer you to see a dietitian.

Glycaemic index (GI)

The glycaemic index (GI) can be used as a guide to measure how quickly foods that contain carbohydrate raise blood glucose levels. The index has been calculated by looking at the rise in blood glucose levels after ingesting 50 grams of carbohydrate contained in individual carbohydrate foods.

High and low GI foods

Foods are given a value of 0 to 100, with glucose being 100. Foods with a GI greater than 70 are classed as high GI foods, so they increase blood glucose quickly; those with a GI of 58 to 69 are classed as medium GI foods and have a moderate effect on blood glucose; those with a GI less than 55 are classed as low GI foods because they have a slow or only minor impact on blood glucose levels.

It seems sensible to follow a low GI diet, but you need to be aware of the following points:

- Foods with a low GI value tend to be high in fibre. They are digested slowly and so lower the GI response; they will have less effect on blood glucose after a meal.

- Foods with a low GI value tend to fill you up for longer, which can be beneficial for weight loss because you may be inclined to eat less.

- There is some evidence to suggest that glycaemic control improves in people who eat foods with a low GI value.

- Low GI foods have been found to increase HDL-cholesterol and lower the total cholesterol and triglyceride levels – a good thing!

- The addition of seeds or grains tends to lower the GI, for example granary bread has a lower GI than wholemeal bread.

- The GI takes into account only single foods. If you eat more than one type of carbohydrate at a time then the GI changes. If high and low GI foods are eaten together, the GI value of the meal will be halfway between the two individual values.

- Cooking and preparation of food can alter the GI value, for example mashed potato (high) or chips (medium). Cooking breaks down the chemical bonds in complex carbohydrates, which makes them easier to absorb and will therefore increase the GI. This does not happen with pulses, however, which have a GI that remains low after cooking. The bonds are also broken when food is chewed, which can therefore raise the GI.

- Highly processed convenience foods tend to have a high GI, for example pastries.

- Ripeness can affect the GI. A ripe banana will have a higher GI than an unripe one.

Some low GI foods are so slowly absorbed, for example pulses/nuts, that insulin may be absorbed more rapidly than digested food. A diet high in these types of foods may predispose to low blood glucose levels (see 'All about hypoglycaemia', page 76).

Fat and protein slow down the absorption of carbohydrate and therefore lower the GI value, for example chips and crisps have a lower GI than potatoes

Glycaemic index of different foods

High glycaemic index
- Glucose
- Instant mashed potato
- Mashed potato
- Jacket potato
- Cornflakes
- Jelly sweets
- White bread

Medium glycaemic index
- Basmati rice
- Honey
- Banana (ripe)
- Boiled potatoes
- Grain bread, e.g. granary

Low glycaemic index
- Banana (unripe)
- Apple
- Lentils
- Nuts

because of their fat content. However, eating low GI foods that are high in fat can lead to weight gain.

As a result of these concerns there may be problems in following a GI diet to the letter, but it is useful to be aware of the GI of foods that you eat regularly. It is sensible to have a low GI food at each mealtime.

Overall it is important to follow a balanced diet, rich in fibre, fruit and vegetables, low in fat and salt, so use any knowledge of GI as part of an overall dietary strategy.

Alcohol

Having diabetes doesn't mean turning teetotal unless you prefer to, but you do have to follow a few commonsense rules, particularly if you are on tablets or insulin. Remember that alcohol can cause hypoglycaemia in certain circumstances (low blood glucose, see page 76).

- Limit yourself to the correct number of 'units' in any one day as shown on page 42. One unit of alcohol means a single measure of spirits, half a pint of beer or a small glass of wine.

- Avoid 'diabetic' or Pils-type beers or lagers because, although they have less sugar, they are high in alcohol and more likely to cause a low blood glucose.

What is a unit of alcohol?

A one-litre bottle of spirits – brandy, whisky or gin – contains about 40 units of alcohol

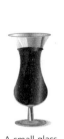 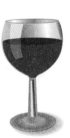 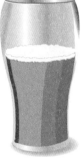

| A small glass of sherry or fortified wine | A standard glass of wine | 1/2 pint of beer or cider 1/2 pint of strong lager | A single measure of aperitif or spirit |

- Drink alcohol with or just after a meal and make sure that you have some slow-release carbohydrate with it. You will need a snack before you go to bed in order to help prevent your blood glucose levels from dropping during the night.

- You may find that your face flushes red if you mix alcohol with some kinds of diabetes tablet treatment.

- Remember to allow for the calorie content of alcoholic drinks and mixers, which should be diet/slimline versions.

Current government recommendations for alcohol intake are as follows:

- 1–2 units per day, 14 units per week for women
- 2–3 units per day, 21 units per week for men
- Always have some alcohol-free days during the week.

KEY POINTS

- Eat regularly

- Include some starchy food (carbohydrate) with each meal, choosing high-fibre versions where possible

- Reduce your fat intake and remember to watch the type of fat

- Limit your intake of sugars and sugary foods

- Aim to keep to your ideal body weight and exercise regularly when possible

- Use salt sparingly

- Do not drink too much alcohol

Treatment: medication

Tablet treatment

There are six main kinds of tablet treatment for people with type 2 diabetes:

1 sulphonylureas

2 biguanides

3 acarbose

4 thiazolidinediones

5 glitinides

6 gliptins.

They all come under the general name of oral hypoglycaemic agents (OHAs), and any of them may be taken alone or in combination. Most people with type 2 diabetes find that these medications, together with a healthy eating pattern, keep their diabetes well under control, although it may take a while to find out which combination or dose suits them best. However, with the passage of time, patients can gradually lose their responsiveness to the tablets and blood glucose levels rise to the extent that insulin injections are needed.

If you do experience side effects or find that your blood glucose levels are higher than they should be, you should go back to your GP to discuss possible changes to your treatment.

Sulphonylureas

Sulphonylureas (SUs) work by stimulating the pancreas to release stored insulin. You could say that they raise the insulin level by proxy, and so help to keep blood glucose down. You have to remember that, although you're not actually taking insulin, these tablets have a similar effect because they increase the amount of insulin in your bloodstream, and it is possible for it to increase too much. If this happens, your blood glucose levels will drop too far, and you may sometimes experience the symptoms of hypoglycaemia (too little glucose in the blood, see page 76). To prevent this happening, you should make sure that you eat regularly, and take your tablets either with or just before a meal.

As with insulin, SUs can be short, medium or long acting (see below), and must be taken once, twice or three times a day depending on how fast they work. The long-acting versions do not always suit older people or those whose lifestyle makes it difficult to have regular mealtimes because of the risk of hypoglycaemia.

Side effects

Apart from having to be aware of the risk of low blood glucose (hypoglycaemia), most people taking SUs find

Names of sulphonylurea tablets available in the UK

All these different kinds of sulphonylurea tablets stimulate the pancreas to release stored insulin, raising the level of insulin and thereby helping to keep blood glucose levels down.

Chemical or generic name	Trade or proprietary name	Duration of action
Chlorpropamide	n/a	Long
Glibenclamide	Daonil/Euglucon	Medium
Gliclazide	Diamicron	Medium
Glimepiride	Amaryl	Medium
Glipizide	Glibenese/Minodiab	Medium
Tolbutamide	n/a	Short

that they have few, if any, serious side effects. Probably the most annoying one is that some patients find that their faces can get very flushed and hot when they drink alcohol. The precise reasons for this side effect are unclear.

As you'll soon discover once you're taking them, the fact that SUs lower your blood glucose will make you feel very hungry so you could gain a lot of weight if you're not careful.

A minority of people won't be able to take SUs because they're allergic to them, and if you're allergic to the antibiotic Septrin you may also have a reaction to SUs.

Biguanides

This type of drug has been in use for over 50 years, and the only one available in this country is metformin. No one is sure precisely how it works, but it seems to slow down the absorption of glucose from the intestines, reducing the blood surge after a meal, and it may also have a more complicated effect on the liver.

As a result of this, you can't take it if you have any kind of liver disease, and it is also best avoided in patients with kidney complications (see page 113). You don't have to worry about your blood glucose level dropping too far when you're on metformin because it doesn't stimulate the release of insulin.

It's often prescribed for people who are overweight because it doesn't make you feel hungry or put on extra pounds. You normally start on a low dose, taking it once or twice a day with meals, and then gradually build up the amount that you're taking as you get used to it.

Side effects

The main side effects are stomach upsets – nausea and diarrhoea – and some people have to stop taking it because of this problem.

Acarbose

This works in quite a different way from the other OHAs. By interfering with the breakdown of carbohydrates in the intestine, it stops your body from absorbing glucose from food.

Unfortunately, this means that more sugars remain unabsorbed in the large intestine where lots of bacteria and micro-organisms lurk. These feed on the abundant sugar and proliferate, which can mean that you suffer from loose motions and flatus (wind). Nevertheless, it could be the right option for you if you find it difficult to follow a healthy eating plan or tend to be overweight.

Thiazolidinediones (glitazones)

Thiazolidinediones increase the sensitivity of cells to the effects of insulin. Rosiglitazone and pioglitazone are licensed for use in the UK. They are usually used with either an SU or metformin and, although they do not cause hypoglycaemia directly, they can produce it in combination with SUs.

The most common side effects are weight gain and fluid retention. Extensive clinical trials are ongoing.

These tablets have been licensed for use on their own and are available in a single-tablet combination with metformin. Scientists reviewing the results of large trials of these medicines have found that they may cause osteoporosis (thinning of the bones) and predispose to fractures. Rosiglitazone has also been linked to heart attacks and some doctors suggest that it should not be used in people with known heart disease.

Glitinides

Two of these tablets are available in the UK (repaglinide and nateglinide). They are taken immediately before meals and lower glucose by stimulating insulin release. However, because of their short action they are thought to be less likely to produce hypoglycaemia than conventional SUs.

Gliptins

Two new drugs, vildagliptin and sitagliptin, are now available. They work by preventing the breakdown of glucagon-like peptide 1 (GLP-1), which is a hormone released by the intestines in response to food. GLP-1 is a powerful stimulant for insulin release from the pancreas. Short-term trials show promising results but longer-term studies are awaited.

Incretins

Research using a form of GLP-1, called exenatide, has found it to be very effective at both lowering blood glucose and losing weight. Its drawback is that it has to be given by injection, twice a day, although a longer-acting weekly preparation is undergoing research. Exenatide is now available in the UK. Its main side effect is stomach upset (nausea and sickness). An alternative preparation called liraglutide, which is a once-daily injection, will soon become available in the UK.

When you need insulin

When you have type 1 diabetes, there's no alternative to replacing the missing insulin by means of daily injections. People whose diabetes is not effectively controlled by diet and tablets may also have to change to insulin injections.

If you've just found this out, it's bound to take you a while to adjust to the idea but, with the right information and back-up from your diabetes care team, you'll soon realise that you will be able to cope and keep yourself well. They will show you how to give injections, and take time to teach you how to manage your condition effectively.

Don't worry if you need to see them several times to get things clear – no one will mind. In fact, they will encourage you to keep asking questions and coming back until you feel comfortable with all the masses of new information. Here are some of the questions that people with newly diagnosed diabetes ask most often.

Why inject the insulin?

This is the only effective way of getting it into your bloodstream. If you swallow it, it is partly digested and so becomes less active, which means that it can't do its job of controlling your blood glucose level. Although other ways of giving insulin have been tried, they've all had problems, so injection is the only practical option for the time being.

Why is insulin injected under the skin?

In theory, it could be injected into a vein or a muscle, as happens with some other medicines such as antibiotics. In practice, however, injecting the insulin into a vein several times a day would be difficult, and intramuscular injections can be painful. Both these methods are sometimes used in special circumstances – for instance when you are ill or can't eat regularly, perhaps because you're having an operation.

What types of insulin are there?

The basic difference is in how quickly they take effect, so that they can be divided into short-, medium- or long-acting varieties. The short-acting insulin is always clear or colourless, whereas the other two are usually cloudy because they contain additives to slow down the absorption of insulin from under the skin. It is possible to mix short- and medium-acting insulins in the same syringe, but care must be taken not to contaminate the clear insulin with any cloudy insulin. For this reason the clear insulin is always drawn up first.

If you find it difficult to mix insulins yourself, you may be able to use one of the ready-mixed kinds that contain quick- and medium-acting insulins in different proportions.

Insulin injections

Injecting insulin is the most effective way to take it, since if taken by mouth insulin is partly destroyed by digestive juices before reaching the bloodstream.

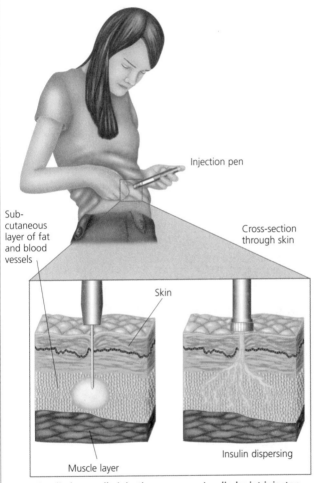

Injection pen

Sub-cutaneous layer of fat and blood vessels

Cross-section through skin

Skin

Insulin dispersing

Muscle layer

Insulin by needle injection
Insulin is released through a needle between the skin and muscle

Insulin by jet injector
Insulin enters the skin under force of pressure

Where does this insulin come from?

All three types of insulin may be produced from animal sources – pig or beef – or from genetically engineered human hormone. Recently, scientists have been able to create modified insulins using the new genetic technology. These insulins, called analogues, are absorbed either more quickly or more slowly and smoothly.

Quick-acting analogues (Humalog or NovoRapid) can be injected immediately before, during or even after a meal, and are therefore more convenient to use, particularly for people with variable mealtimes. They also enable you to have a bit more insulin if the meal was larger than expected.

The only long-acting analogues available in the UK at the moment are glargine and detemir. These insulins can be given once or twice daily at any time but preferably at the same time each day. Unlike other long-acting insulins, glargine and detemir are clear solutions and care must be taken not to confuse them with fast-acting preparations.

Detailed research trials are ongoing to discover the best way of using these new insulins, but early results suggest that analogues may be associated with less hypoglycaemia.

Is human insulin better than pig or beef?

This is a controversial area and some patients who changed from animal to human insulin have said that they feel less well since the switch. It seems that human insulin is absorbed slightly more quickly from under the skin.

However, no measurable differences in blood glucose levels have been found when human and animal insulins were tested under control conditions, but some people do prefer the animal preparations. At the moment supplies are still available and said to be guaranteed for the foreseeable future.

Why do I have to inject insulin several times a day?

The object of insulin therapy is to imitate the body's natural supply as closely as possible. In a person who doesn't have diabetes, insulin is released by the pancreas in response to food (see diagram on page 56). As the blood glucose level falls between meals, so the insulin level drops back towards zero. It never quite gets there, however, and there is no time in the 24 hours when there is no detectable insulin in the bloodstream. What you are trying to do when you give yourself insulin injections is to reproduce the normal pattern of insulin production from the pancreas.

There are several ways of doing this using different types of insulin and numbers of injections per day. For example, many people follow a system of injections of short-acting insulin before the three main meals of the day, plus a night-time injection of a medium- or long-acting insulin to control blood glucose while they're asleep.

Another popular and equally successful system involves two injections a day of a mixture of short- and medium-acting insulins. The idea is that the short-acting component covers the meal that you're about to have (say breakfast or tea/evening meal), while the medium-acting component covers you at lunchtime or overnight. Many people have been using one or other of these systems very happily for years, and the choice between them is often simply a matter of personal preference.

If you're one of the relatively few people who simply can't get used to giving themselves several injections a day, or if you have only a partial failure of your insulin supply, you may be able to make do with just one or two daily injections of medium- or long-acting insulin.

How and where do I inject myself?

Your diabetes care team will show you how to do the injections and explain the various types of equipment available. Most people today use disposable plastic syringes and needles.

Needle and syringe

Injection by needle and syringe continues to be a popular way to administer insulin.

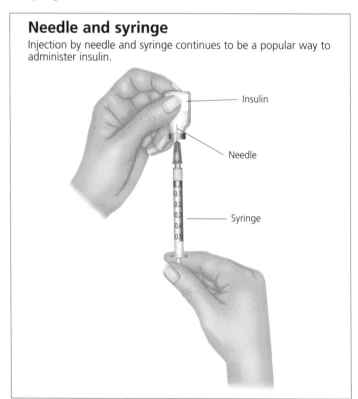

Insulin

Needle

Syringe

Disposable syringes and needles can be used several times with little risk of infection. They are usually thrown away when the needle becomes blunt and injections become less comfortable.

Insulin injection pens are very popular, largely because of their convenience and portability. The pens themselves and the needles are available on prescription. There are several types of pen to choose from, but the principles of the device are much the same. It's simply a matter of which one suits you best.

As we've already seen, you inject insulin under your skin rather than into a vein or muscle. Recent research has suggested that many people may have been getting the depth wrong so that insulin is going into the muscle beneath the skin by mistake.

Insulin pen

Many people prefer to use insulin pens rather than the more traditional syringes and needles. Insulin pens are simple to use and can be carried around easily.

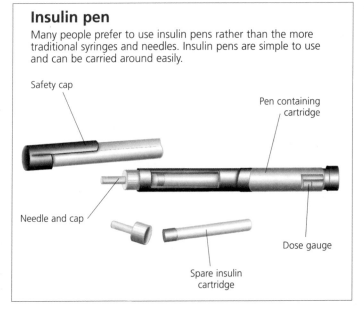

Safety cap

Pen containing cartridge

Needle and cap

Dose gauge

Spare insulin cartridge

Levels of insulin and blood glucose

These graphs of the levels of glucose and insulin in the blood show the normal pattern of insulin release, and the way in which insulin injections relate to mealtimes.

Normal pattern of insulin release

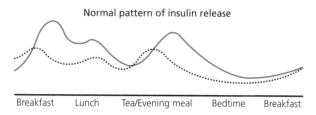

| Breakfast | Lunch | Tea/Evening meal | Bedtime | Breakfast |

Insulin release with multiple injections

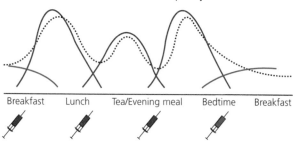

| Breakfast | Lunch | Tea/Evening meal | Bedtime | Breakfast |

Insulin release with twice daily injections

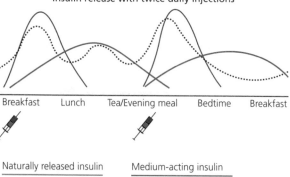

| Breakfast | Lunch | Tea/Evening meal | Bedtime | Breakfast |

Naturally released insulin   Medium-acting insulin

Short-acting insulin   Blood glucose

Levels of insulin and blood glucose (contd)

Description of treatment regime

Natural insulin release
In a person who does not have diabetes, insulin is released by the pancreas in response to the rise in blood glucose levels produced by eating food. Glucose levels are kept within a tight range.

Insulin injections before meals and before bedtime (basal–bolus)
To reproduce normal conditions, many people inject themselves with short-acting insulin three times a day before meals, plus a night-time injection of medium- or long-acting insulin to control blood glucose overnight. Mealtimes are flexible with this method.

Two types of insulin injected twice daily
Two injections a day of both short- and medium-acting insulins cover the meal that you are about to have as well as a later meal or overnight. Timing of meals is important to avoid low glucose levels.

Judging the depth accurately can be quite difficult, especially if you're slim, but it's important to master the technique because insulin can be absorbed from muscle more rapidly than expected.

Your diabetes care team will show you how to do it properly, but a lot of people find that the simplest way is to inject at an angle of 90 degrees. There is a range of different length pen needles now available so it is easier to control the depth of injections. It is important for you to find the right type of needle depending on your injection site and body size. This needs to be discussed with your diabetes care team.

You'll be given advice about the best sites for injection (see figure opposite). The tops of the thighs, buttocks and abdomen are the most common sites, and it's best to avoid using the same area every time, otherwise you could develop a small fatty lump (called lipohypertrophy) which could affect the smoothness of insulin absorption.

It's probably a good idea to inject medium- or longer-acting insulins into your thigh or buttock and use your tummy for quick-acting injections, but the most important thing is that you should be happy about the sites that you're using.

Will the injections hurt?

People who've been giving themselves injections for years say that they don't feel a thing, but many beginners may find it slightly painful at first. Try to be as relaxed as you can and follow the technique that you've been shown. Some people find that it helps to rub the skin with ice for a few seconds beforehand to numb it, and you might like to give this a try.

As you get more practice, you should find that the injections rarely hurt, but, if things don't improve, it's

Insulin injection sites

The thighs, abdomen and buttocks are the main sites in which to inject insulin.

Abdomen
Absorbs insulin quckly – don't inject close to the tummy button

Arms
Absorb insulin more slowly than the abdomen

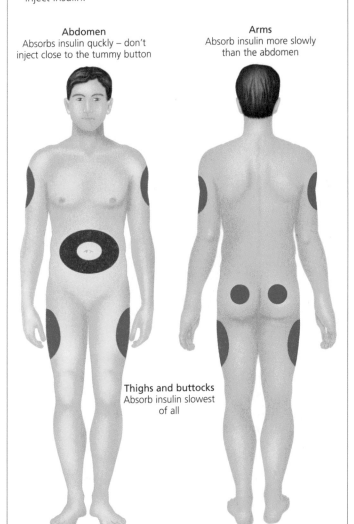

Thighs and buttocks
Absorb insulin slowest of all

worth asking someone at the diabetes care centre for advice on what's causing the problem.

Will the injections leave a mark?

The needles are very fine and usually do not leave a mark. Sometimes you may get a little bleeding after an injection or even a bruise, but this is nothing to worry about. It just means that you've probably punctured one of the tiny blood vessels under the skin, and this happens from time to time. There is virtually no chance of insulin directly entering the bloodstream, so don't worry if you notice some bleeding.

Can you give insulin by other routes?

Until recently, inhaled insulin was available. It required a rather large device, which was much bigger than an asthma inhaler. Insulin given this way is no more effective than by injection, and you would still need to inject overnight insulin because only short-acting preparations can be inhaled.

Although there have been no safety concerns so far, long-term effects on the lungs cannot be completely ruled out. Finally, inhaled insulin was wasteful, needing 10 times the dose used by injection, and it was expensive. It was probably most useful if you were needle phobic and could not contemplate injections, and definitely needed insulin for your diabetes control. Unfortunately the only supplier has recently withdrawn its product from the UK.

Can you take insulin and tablets at the same time?

Some type 2 patients who need insulin and are also insulin resistant can benefit from a combination of

Insulin pump therapy

An insulin pump delivers a continuous infusion of insulin through a tube (catheter) that is placed underneath the skin on the abdomen. The pump delivers a variable but constant background insulin dose. Patients give top-up doses or 'boluses' at meal times. Carbohydrate counting (see page 23) is an essential part of pump use.

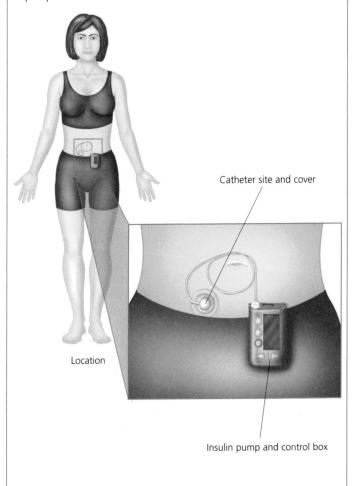

Catheter site and cover

Location

Insulin pump and control box

injections and metformin. Increasingly, doctors prescribe a combination of long-acting insulin and an SU or glitinide before meals.

What about an insulin pump?

Some patients have found that giving insulin by a constant infusion under the skin via a thin plastic tube and needle gives smoother blood glucose control. Pumps therefore require a lot of input from the patients who use them. They may be particularly effective in young children who struggle with multiple injections. Pumps are expensive (around £2,800) and cost more than £1,000 every year to run. They also require considerable medical expertise as back-up.

The National Institute for Health and Clinical Excellence (NICE; see 'Useful addresses', page 149) has approved insulin pump therapy for patients with type 1 diabetes who find it difficult to achieve satisfactory blood glucose control without experiencing hypoglycaemia. Their advice was revised in 2008 and is available on the website.

Specialised diabetes units have been set up around the UK. Funding should now be available. To check the situation in your district, contact your diabetes care team.

It is hoped that the 'postcode lottery' for pumps should soon become a thing of the past.

KEY POINTS

■ Tablet treatment is useful for type 2 patients

■ Tablets work in different ways and have different side effects. Be sure to check these with your diabetes care team when they are prescribed

■ Insulin injections are necessary for all patients with type 1 and many with type 2 diabetes

■ At least two and maybe four injections of insulin are needed a day

■ Injections rarely cause discomfort or leave any mark

■ Insulin preparations can be short, medium or long acting

■ Pre-mixed short- and medium-acting preparations are now available

■ A combination of insulin and tablets may suit some patients with type 2 diabetes

■ Insulin pumps are increasingly available and may be particularly useful for children or those with troublesome hypoglycaemia (see page 76)

Checking your glucose levels

The objective of diabetes treatment

The point of all treatment for diabetes – whether it's diet, tablets or insulin – is to keep the levels of glucose in your bloodstream as close as possible to normal. The nearer you get to achieving this, the better you will feel, especially in the long term.

Blood glucose monitoring

There are two ways in which you can monitor glucose levels for yourself and your diabetes team will advise you about which one you should use and how often to do the checks. The two methods available are:

1 blood tests

2 urine tests

and neither is particularly difficult once you get the hang of it.

The development of simple fingerprick blood testing methods in the last few years has transformed life for patients taking insulin. Keeping a close check on your glucose levels is very useful when you're on insulin because it means that you can make adjustments to your dose depending on the results.

When your diabetes is being controlled by tablets and/or diet, urine tests can give you almost as much information as blood tests and may be more convenient. Recent evidence suggests little or no benefit of blood glucose tests in patients with type 2 diabetes on diet or oral hypoglycaemic agents.

In addition, there are blood tests that measure an average blood glucose level over a period before the test – from two to eight weeks. Each of these three approaches is looked at in turn.

Blood tests

There are two systems available for self-blood glucose monitoring (or SBGM as you may hear it called). Both give accurate results and, as well as helping you improve your blood glucose control, they can be useful if you suspect that you may be about to have a hypoglycaemic reaction (see page 76).

Taking an exact reading will either reassure you that all is well or confirm that you need to take action. Blood testing strips are available on prescription but the special meters for reading them may have to be purchased separately, although many diabetes centres are able to offer them for free.

Method 1

The glucose in the drop of your blood reacts with a pad or pads on the end of a plastic strip. These pads have been impregnated with chemicals and form colours when exposed to glucose. The strip is inserted into the appropriate meter, which gives a reading.

There are several different strips available, each of which has a different reaction time, so it is vital to follow the manufacturer's instructions carefully.

Method 2

A slightly more complicated chemical reaction takes place when a drop of your blood is put on the specially designed testing strip. There is no colour change involved and the strips can be read only using a special meter. This system needs slightly less blood than the conventional colour pad system.

It is now possible to measure both blood glucose and ketones using a fingerprick test and a special strip and meter. This technique may be particularly useful in pregnancy and in young people who are prone to recurrent episodes of ketoacidosis.

How to do the test

The main drawback for some people is that both these systems mean that you have to obtain a fingerprick sample of your own blood (although occasionally someone else may be able to do this for you).

Pricking your finger can be especially difficult if you are a manual worker or if you have very sensitive fingers. Rather than having to nerve yourself deliberately to stab your finger, you might find it easier to use one of the devices incorporating a spring-loaded lancet (needle). It allows you to adjust the depth of the prick to suit yourself, but the disadvantage is that, although the lancets are available on prescription, the spring-loaded devices sometimes have to be paid for.

Testing blood to determine the glucose level

A blood sample must first be obtained which is dabbed on to a testing strip. The strip is placed into a special meter to give a very precise blood glucose reading.

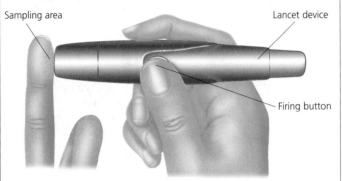

Sampling area

Lancet device

Firing button

1. Prick the side of your finger using the spring-loaded lancet

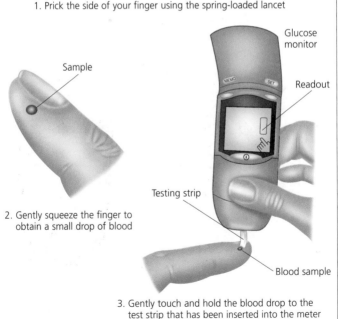

Sample

Glucose monitor

Readout

Testing strip

Blood sample

2. Gently squeeze the finger to obtain a small drop of blood

3. Gently touch and hold the blood drop to the test strip that has been inserted into the meter

Examples of blood glucose meters

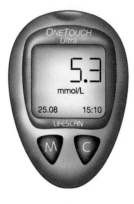

One Touch Ultra

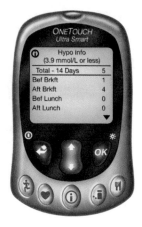

One Touch UltraSmart

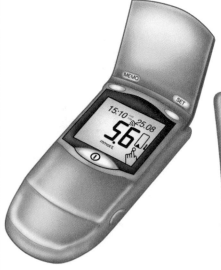

Accu-Chek Compact

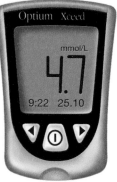

Optium Xceed

Glucose sensors
Devices implanted in the body

These use a fine needle that is placed under the skin, usually on the abdomen or tummy. This needle is connected via a fine tube to a small device worn on a belt or on the abdomen. Special enzymes on the needle break down glucose in the fluid under the skin and this creates a small electric current, which is detected by the device and converted into a glucose level. The results are stored and downloaded into a computer after three to five days or transmitted 'real time' to give an immediate result.

A similar device using a different method has also been developed. A small pump pushes fluid under the skin, which absorbs glucose from the tissue. This fluid is then returned back into the device and the glucose concentration is measured. This system can measure glucose levels for up to two days.

These machines can be useful to detect patterns of glucose control and provide a basis for treatment changes. Recently, they have been connected to an insulin pump so that indications can be made for dosage as well as warnings for hypoglycaemia. These devices are not yet available on the NHS and are awaiting assessment from NICE.

Newer devices measure glucose levels every three minutes and show the readings on a small screen – so-called 'real time'. They are currently rather expensive and are undergoing further intensive research. An exciting development has been the linking of these systems to an insulin pump and, by using a small computer chip, the device recommends insulin doses to the patient before meals.

Infrared devices

A non-invasive method uses an infrared light shone across small blood vessels. The level of glucose in the blood will affect the impedance of the light across the vessel and generate a signal, which can be converted to provide a blood glucose value. This method is, however, still highly experimental.

Urine tests
Kidney (or renal) threshold for glucose reabsorption

Glucose appears in your urine when your kidneys can no longer reabsorb the amount being filtered. The problem with urine testing is that this 'overflow point' isn't the same for everyone. The correct term for this overflow point is the kidney (or renal) threshold for glucose reabsorption.

Some people who don't have diabetes have a low threshold, and they often need the glucose tolerance test, described on page 16, to confirm the fact and explain why glucose has appeared in their urine.

The normal threshold is around a blood glucose level of 10 millimoles per litre (mmol/l) so, for a person with diabetes, a negative urine test can mean that your blood glucose level is anywhere between 0 and 10 mmol/l, depending on your personal threshold. A positive test, on the other hand, doesn't tell you the exact level of blood glucose or by how much it exceeds your own personal threshold.

Despite this relative lack of accuracy, however, testing your urine and getting mostly negative results may be all you need to confirm that you have your diabetes well under control, especially if you're being treated with diet and/or tablets.

Kidney threshold for glucose reabsorption

The kidneys can only reabsorb a certain level of glucose, typically 10 mmol/l. If this level is exceeded, as it may be if blood glucose levels are out of control, glucose appears in the urine.

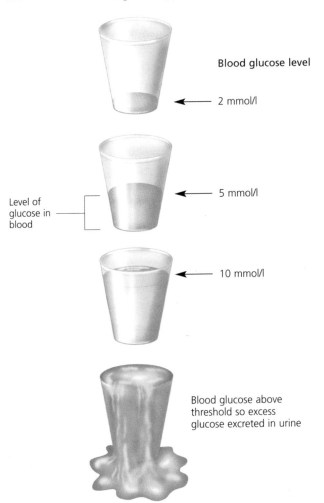

Blood glucose level

2 mmol/l

Level of glucose in blood

5 mmol/l

10 mmol/l

Blood glucose above threshold so excess glucose excreted in urine

How to do the test

Nearly everyone these days uses stick tests similar to those used for testing blood glucose. You dip a stick either into the stream of urine or into a specimen that you've just passed, wait for the chemical reaction that results in a colour change, and then read off the colour against the chart, which is usually printed on the side of the container.

As with the blood testing sticks, how long you wait varies from one type of urine stick to another, so do check the manufacturer's instructions.

The test must be done on fresh urine if it is to reflect the level of glucose in your blood at the time that it's done. This is especially important first thing in the morning, when urine may have been accumulating in your bladder over several hours.

What you have to do is empty your bladder about half an hour before you want to do the test, then pass another sample about half an hour later which is the one that you actually check.

Urine stick tests

Device for checking colour on urine stick tests.

| | neg. | 0,1 (5,5) | 0,25 (14) | 0,5 (28) | 1 (56) | 2 (111) | 3 (167) | 5% (280) (mmol/l) %=g/dL |

What the results of blood or urine tests show

When you do either a blood or a urine test, you're really measuring how effective your previous dose of insulin or tablet treatment has been. In other words, doing a test just before lunch will tell someone on insulin the effect of the early morning injection of quick-acting insulin. In the same way, a pre-breakfast test will reflect the effectiveness of the previous night-time dose. The same interpretation applies in principle to tablets.

Adjusting doses

When the test result shows a high level of glucose, you may have to increase the size of your next dose of medication to restore the balance. This solves the problem short term, but ideally you want to prevent the problem arising in the first place by adjusting the dose that preceded the test.

It's a good idea to vary the time of day when you do your test, and also to wait for a series of results over a period of, say, three to five days, before making too many adjustments. That way, you will see whether there is any pattern to the changes in your blood glucose level.

Until you have more experience of handling your diabetes, it would be better to consult your GP or someone in your diabetes care team before altering your insulin or tablet dosage. Later on, once you've learned more about your body's reactions, you'll be able to make the necessary adjustments on your own because you'll know what works for you.

Clinic monitoring

There may be situations where your medical advisers feel that it would be useful to assess the effectiveness of your treatment by means of more sophisticated blood tests. They are not a substitute for your own routine testing, but can give additional information, which will help your diabetes care team decide whether your treatment needs adjustment. Both tests usually require a blood sample to be taken from a vein, although some new machines use only a fingerprick blood sample.

Glycated haemoglobin

This is a test that measures your average blood glucose level over a period of some six to eight weeks. It is reported as a percentage, unlike blood glucose (units of millimoles per litre or mmol/l), and the normal (non-diabetic) range is usually between four and six per cent.

Good control is usually defined as a value of 7.5 per cent or less; poor control is 10 per cent or more. Roughly speaking, a glycated haemoglobin of 7.5 per cent is equivalent to an average blood glucose of 10 mmol/l, whereas a value of 10 per cent is equivalent to an average of 15 mmol/l. Like all averages, however, it could be the result of lots of small variations or much larger swings in either direction. For this reason, this test isn't useful for making day-to-day adjustments of insulin treatment, but is a good guide as to whether your treatment is working well overall.

Fructosamine

This test works on the same principle as glycated

haemoglobin, but measures treatment effectiveness over a shorter period – about two to three weeks. Again it is a useful guide as to whether your current treatment is working well or needs adjustment.

KEY POINTS

■ Blood tests provide accurate information about glucose control

■ Blood tests are helpful to exclude hypoglycaemia (low blood glucose)

■ Urine tests are perfectly adequate for monitoring patients on diet control or low doses of oral hypoglycaemic agents (OHAs), but are not very helpful for alerting the patient to hypoglycaemia

All about hypoglycaemia

Who is affected?

You need to be concerned about 'hypos' only if you are being treated with insulin, a sulphonylurea (SU) or glitinide tablets. If your diabetes is controlled just by diet or you are taking metformin, thiazolidinediones or acarbose, you will not experience this problem.

What is hypoglycaemia?

Hypoglycaemia means low blood glucose and, in a person who doesn't have diabetes, the levels never fall much below 3.5 millimoles per litre (mmol/l). This is because their natural control system will sense the drop, and correct the situation by stopping insulin secretion and releasing other hormones such as glucagon, which boost blood glucose. What's more, the person will start to feel hungry, and so do the right thing by eating, so raising the blood glucose.

When you're on insulin or SUs, this feedback system no longer operates. Once you have taken

Symptoms of hypoglycaemia

You should be aware of the symptoms of hypoglycaemia, so that you can take appropriate action. Frequent 'hypos' may indicate that your treatment or eating pattern needs adjusting.

- Feeling sweaty or cold and clammy
- Trembling and feeling weak
- Tingling around your lips
- Feeling hungry
- Blurred vision
- Feeling irritable, upset or angry
- Unable to concentrate
- Looking pale
- Feeling drowsy (and losing consciousness if nothing is done)

Sometimes, people with low blood glucose levels may behave oddly, so that others may suspect them of being drunk.

Most people who are taking insulin can use their symptoms as a signal that they need to have some food fairly quickly.

However, just which symptoms you get and how severe they are is an individual thing – some people feel hungry before noticing anything else; others experience tingling round the lips or shakiness, for example.

You may not experience all of these symptoms, but it is usual to have a headache after a 'hypo'.

Reaction times may be prolonged for several hours after experiencing a hypoglycaemic reaction. Patients should not drive or undertake hazardous activities during this time.

insulin or stimulated its production with tablets, you
can't switch it off again, so your blood glucose will go
on dropping until you have some food in the form of
carbohydrate.

As the level falls, it usually triggers a variety of
warning symptoms (see box on page 77).
Hypoglycaemia is dangerous because the brain
depends almost entirely on glucose for normal
functioning. If levels drop too low, it starts to work less
well and produces the symptoms shown in the box.
If the level drops even lower, unconsciousness (coma)
may result.

Preventing hypos

In past years, someone who was being started on
insulin might have had to go through a deliberately
induced hypoglycaemic reaction so that he or she
would know how it felt. These days your doctor is
unlikely to suggest this because it's not very pleasant!

Doing a blood glucose test yourself means that you
can find out quickly and easily whether your level is
getting too low and take action if necessary.

One of the most important aspects of caring for
patients with diabetes is trying to ensure that they
don't suffer from hypoglycaemic reactions. This
involves the individual concerned discussing treatment
and adjusting it if necessary to fit in with his or her
lifestyle, especially with mealtimes and work patterns.
This is not always easy, and sometimes it means
compromises will have to be worked out.

You usually have to accept that there is no
alternative to sticking to regular mealtimes, however
inconvenient you find it. With the wide range of
different insulins and types of injection device, it is

usually possible, however, to arrive at a treatment programme that will suit you.

Having regular hypoglycaemic attacks is a sign that you need to go back to your doctor or nurse to see how your treatment and/or eating pattern can be adjusted to prevent them happening.

What causes hypos?

You'll soon get to recognise the situations where you are especially vulnerable, but the most common are:

- Eating later than you had expected or planned, which is bound to happen sometimes. If you've had your insulin injection and then can't eat for some reason, you should eat a small carbohydrate snack (such as a boiled sweet or a biscuit), which you ought to have handy at all times.

- A burst of unexpected exercise – such as running for a bus (for more on this, see page 86).

- Drinking too much alcohol. When your liver has to break down excessive quantities of alcohol, it can't produce glucose at the same time. This is why you'll be advised not to drink too much alcohol if you're on insulin or taking SUs or glitinides. Always eat something whenever you do have an alcoholic drink.

Treating a hypo

A reaction that's relatively mild can usually be dealt with quite simply – a glass of Lucozade or lemonade should do the trick. Remember, however, that diet drinks contain artificial sweetener rather than sugar, so are of no use to you in this situation.

Do make sure, too, that, wherever you are, you always carry some sort of readily available carbohydrate in the form of a boiled sweet or biscuit. Chocolate is not very useful in this situation because it is a slow-release form of carbohydrate. Having readily available carbohydrate is especially important if you're a driver or if you're about to take some form of vigorous exercise. For more on this, see the sections on diet (page 18) and exercise (page 86).

Severe hypos

Very occasionally, you may find that your blood glucose level drops so rapidly that you don't have time to take the corrective action described above. You may become drowsy or unconscious, and might even have an epileptic fit.

This is obviously a frightening prospect both for you and for those close to you, and you need to take action to make sure that it doesn't happen again. This means getting advice from your medical team to get the problem sorted out. There are various ways of dealing with a person who's having a severe hypo:

- When you're not in a state to eat or drink anything, a sugary gel called Glucogel or Hypostop can be squirted into your mouth or rubbed on your gums. This should not be done if you are having a fit.

- A hormone called glucagon, which causes blood glucose to rise, is available in injectable form. You can be given an injection into your arm or buttocks to bring you round, so you can then have something to eat or drink. Glucagon should not be used if hypoglycaemia is the result of SU or glitinide treatment, or alcohol intoxication.

Night-time hypos

It's natural for you and your family to worry that you might have a hypo while you're asleep, or even that you might have one and not wake up. This is an especially frightening prospect when you are the parent of a small child with type 1 diabetes – for more on this, see page 100.

In reality, the problem is by no means as dramatic as that. First, you are quite likely to be woken up by the symptoms of falling blood glucose. You may feel sweaty, restless or irritable. Occasionally, your restlessness may wake your partner even if you stay asleep.

It's not unusual to sleep right through a severe hypoglycaemic reaction. Your body mobilises various hormones in response to the falling level of glucose, which stimulates the release of stored glucose to correct the situation. After a reaction like this, you would wake up with a headache and symptoms much like a bad hangover.

Sometimes, there may be a swing too far in the opposite direction, so that your blood glucose rises too high. If you regularly wake up feeling bad with these sort of symptoms it's a good idea to take a few early morning (2 to 4am) blood glucose tests to see if you are having hypoglycaemic reactions that you're not aware of at the time. At least then you'll know why you're feeling so bad and you can talk to your diabetes care team about whether your night-time dose of insulin needs adjusting or altering to a different type.

Losing your hypoglycaemic awareness

You may well have read various stories about some people with diabetes complaining that they have lost their 'early warning system' of a hypoglycaemic

Having a hypo

In hypoglycaemia a low level of glucose in the blood deprives the brain of its source of energy. This condition can occur in diabetes sufferers who are on insulin or SU tablets.

Possible causes:

- A delayed or missed meal or snack
- More exercise than usual – including things like gardening, strenuous housework or sport
- An illness that means you eat less than usual

Treatment:

1 Take some quick-acting carbohydrate, such as glucose tablets or a glucose drink
2 As soon after as you can, have some slower-acting carbohydrate such as sandwiches or toast
3 Check your blood glucose if possible
4 Take more glucose if your symptoms persist
5 If you're due to have a meal or a snack, eat something as soon as you can
6 If your symptoms still don't go, seek medical advice

reaction. Many of them believe that this has happened as a result of changing from animal to human insulin. Before we consider this aspect, we should look at other reasons why this awareness might be lost.

It has become increasingly clear for some years that people who have had diabetes for a very long time become less able to predict when they are about to have a hypo. The warning signs seem to become less noticeable after they've been on insulin for about 15 to 20 years. Although no one knows quite why this should be so, it is true that the ability of the pancreas to release glucagon in response to low blood glucose diminishes over time. Some people say that their symptoms change, whereas others say that the symptoms come on so much faster that they don't have time to take corrective action.

The problem is also more common in people whose average blood glucose levels are on the low side of normal. Sometimes, adjusting the treatment so as to allow the blood glucose level to rise slightly may mean that the person gets the old pattern of symptoms back, but any change of this kind must be discussed carefully with the diabetes care team. Diabetes UK has suggested 'four is the floor', that is, they recommend that blood glucose levels should not be allowed to drop below 4 mmol/l.

Is human insulin to blame?

The question of what role human insulin may play in changing hypoglycaemic awareness is even more complex. Although some patients feel that changing from animal insulin is responsible for their difficulties, their doctors often disagree. Carefully controlled experiments have shown no measurable difference in hypoglycaemic symptoms in people taking animal or human insulin. All the same, some people are quite sure that they feel better on animal insulin and, if so, there is absolutely no reason why they shouldn't go on taking it.

Can hypoglycaemia be avoided by constant high blood glucose levels?

Having persistently high blood glucose levels will avoid hypoglycaemia, but unfortunately this also increases the risk of developing complications of diabetes (see page 107).

Maintaining the balance between risky hyperglycaemia (too much) and troublesome hypoglycaemia (too little) can be very difficult for patients on insulin, but is much easier these days with the different preparations and injection devices available.

If you are having troublesome hypo attacks, followed by high blood glucose levels, consult your diabetes care team because it may mean that your treatment needs adjusting or changing. It may also be worth considering insulin pump treatment (see pages 61–2).

KEY POINTS

■ Hypoglycaemia can occur in any patient taking insulin or sulphonylurea (SU) tablets

■ Individual patients differ in their warning signs of hypoglycaemia

■ If you think a hypo may be coming on, try to confirm with a blood test first

■ If this is not possible take some fast-acting carbohydrate such as Lucozade, lemonade (not low calorie) or glucose tablets

■ Milk and chocolate biscuits are not ideal because they are not rapidly absorbed, but can be useful after initial correction

■ If hypoglycaemia is a recurrent problem, seek advice from your diabetes care team

Breaking your routine

Exercise

When a person who doesn't have diabetes takes exercise, the release of insulin from the pancreas is shut down, whereas other hormones are produced that cause the blood glucose level to rise.

When you're taking insulin or sulphonylurea (SU) tablets, however, your insulin level goes on rising and, if you've had an injection into one of the limbs that you're exercising, the insulin may be absorbed faster than usual.

It's important to let the people you're with – say, your tennis partner or the other members of a football team – know when you're taking insulin and explain to them what to do if you have a hypoglycaemic reaction.

When you know you're going to exercise, you can adjust your medication and/or diet to make allowances. Your dose of insulin may have to be cut by as much as half, depending on how vigorous an exercise session you're planning.

It's more difficult when you take exercise unexpectedly, and this can be a particular problem with children. Once again, the solution is to have your quick-acting carbohydrate snack handy – a sugary drink, a biscuit or glucose tablets.

Hypos

It's important to let the people you're with know when you're taking insulin and explain to them what to do if you have a hypo.

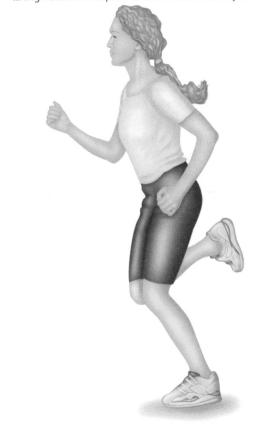

Watch out for delayed hypos

Vigorous exercise can also lead to a delayed
hypoglycaemic reaction. For example, a strenuous
workout in the evening may cause night-time blood
glucose levels to fall as your muscles replenish
glycogen stores. A reduction in the bedtime insulin
dose may be necessary in these circumstances.

Don't stop exercising

As long as you take sensible precautions, there's no
reason at all why you shouldn't take part in any kind
of sport that you want to and at any level. Both Gary
Mabbutt and Alan Kernaghan had type 1 diabetes and
played Premier League football, and Sir Steven
Redgrave – five times Olympic rowing champion –
developed type 1 diabetes before his last gold medal.

Many people with diabetes take part in just about
every known sport – although there are some that
require special considerations, such as scuba diving or
hang gliding, and they might be better avoided! In any
case, the high-risk sports often have special rules and
regulations relating to people with diabetes, and it is
important for your own safety that you abide by them.

Partying

With a little thought and pre-planning, you can feel
free to go to any party and enjoy yourself as much as
ever. The main considerations are that you will
probably be eating later than usual, having different
kinds of food and possibly dancing late into the night.
When you're on insulin, you will need to make certain
adjustments to take account of these factors. When
you know you're going to be having a meal several

Some simple tips for enjoying a night out

There is no need for patients with diabetes to avoid social occasions and parties. Simply follow the commonsense rules below:

- When you're treated with insulin or sulphonylureas, you'll need to eat more to allow for extra activities such as dancing

- Never drink alcohol on an empty stomach; always have some carbohydrate first

- Keep some quick-acting carbohydrate with you on a crowded dance floor in case of hypoglycaemia – it may not be possible to get to a bar or eating area quickly enough

hours later than normal, have a light snack before you go, then delay your injection until the food is ready.

If the party starts really late, you'll probably need extra carbohydrate with your meal along with your normal insulin dose. Take some extra food with you – and perhaps some Lucozade too – if you plan to keep going into the small hours.

The best plan for those on a basal-bolus regime is to substitute the overnight medium-acting insulin with a smaller dose of quick-acting insulin plus a snack at around midnight.

A blood test around three or four hours later is a good idea if you can manage it. Dancing will mean that you have to have extra carbohydrate – how much depends on how much energy you put into your performance!

Travelling

There's no reason why your diabetes should interfere with or restrict your travel plans in any way, although, if you're going abroad, you'd be wise to take out comprehensive travel insurance. Medical care and treatment abroad are rarely free, although the UK does have reciprocal arrangements with some other countries.

If you're going to one of the countries of the European Union, before you go you should obtain a European Heath Insurance Card (EHIC) either by filling in an EHIC form from your post office or by applying online on the Department of Health website (see page 146). Even when a country does offer a reciprocal scheme, it's still worth having your own insurance on top, and essential in those countries where the health care is not equivalent to that provided by the NHS or is very expensive (the USA, for instance).

There may be special considerations when you're heading somewhere extremely remote or inaccessible, so discuss your plans with your diabetes care team. Wherever you're going, and especially if it's off the beaten track, make sure that you will be able to obtain insulin or tablets there if necessary, just in case you somehow get parted from your own supplies. Never pack your insulin in your suitcase! It is a good idea to tell your travel agent or airline that you have diabetes.

You'll need to check out the immunisation requirements for your destination well in advance – sometimes it takes several weeks to complete the course. Preventive measures of this kind may be particularly important for travellers with diabetes, and it is reassuring to know that taking antimalarial tablets will not interfere with treatment for diabetes.

Crossing time zones

You need to plan carefully if you're going on a long flight, and it's a good idea to do this with the help of your doctor or diabetes care team. Remember that travelling west extends your day, whereas travelling east shortens it.

When you're on insulin

You will have fewer problems if you're on a multiple basal-bolus regime using an injection pen than if you normally inject just twice a day. For an extended day, the simplest solution is to have an extra injection of quick-acting insulin before the extra meal that's almost bound to be given during your flight.

When you reach your destination, have your normal evening dose of insulin followed by your evening meal. Next morning, have your insulin before breakfast as usual, then try to match your eating pattern to that of the locals, although this isn't always easy if you have jet lag!

The night will probably be shorter when you're travelling east, so you should have a smaller dose of medium-acting insulin (perhaps 10 to 20 per cent less than usual), either before your evening meal if you're on twice-daily injections or before bed if you're on multiple injections, followed by your usual pre-breakfast dose next day.

Don't forget that you're not obliged to eat all the meals offered on the flight if you feel that you don't want or need them. It is important to let the airline staff know that you have diabetes, and make sure that they or your travelling companions know what to do if you have a hypoglycaemic reaction and how to give insulin if you need it. The same applies if you're travelling by sea.

You don't have to have a fridge to store your insulin as long as you can keep it somewhere relatively cool, but, if temperature is likely to be a problem, use a wide-necked vacuum flask. Do not store insulin in a freezer compartment.

When you're on tablets

You shouldn't need to make any particular changes to your treatment schedule. It would be worth getting the advice of your diabetes care team before taking a very long flight, however, because if you are taking short-acting tablets before meals you may need either an extra one or perhaps one less depending on whether you are flying east or west. The principles are the same for those who are on insulin injections.

Prepare for your journey

You will have to find room in your hand luggage for your medication, blood glucose testing equipment and any other medical kit; luggage does sometimes go missing! When you're carrying syringes and needles, it's sometimes useful to have a letter from your doctor on headed paper explaining that you have diabetes and how it is treated. This is important if you're going to some Middle and Far Eastern countries.

It's also advisable for anyone with diabetes to carry some form of ID card or bracelet indicating that you have the condition and what medication you take. Diabetes UK (see page 147) can supply ID cards giving details of your treatment in the local language of the country that you're going to, and it's worth getting one of these. You may never need to show them, but it won't hurt to have them, just in case.

MedicAlert

MedicAlert Foundation offer an emergency medical information service 24 hours a day. See 'Useful addresses', page 148.

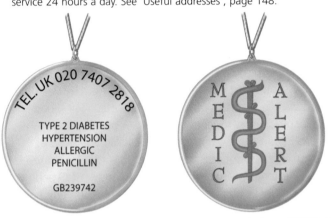

It's quite safe to take travel sickness remedies along with your diabetes treatment if you need to, but, if you know you're prone to suffer in this way, take a supply of fruit juice or other sweet drink in case you can't eat much.

In other respects, you need only to follow the same commonsense rules as any other traveller – make sure that you don't have too much sun, check out the alcohol content of unfamiliar local drinks and try to steer clear of unhygienic cafés or foodstalls!

Take particular care in countries known to have a high risk of water-borne stomach infections. Avoid iced drinks and any fruit or vegetables that you cannot peel, and salads. Use bottled water or drinks wherever possible.

When you are ill

Everyone gets colds and flu from time to time, and these, like other illnesses, can affect the control of your diabetes. The most likely result is that your blood glucose level will rise, so you need to make frequent checks to test whether this is happening, especially if you are on insulin.

Type 1

Many people think that if they're ill and not eating they shouldn't take their insulin, because they will have a hypo. In fact, the opposite is the case. Your blood glucose level is much more likely to be too high than too low in these circumstances. Even if you have a stomach bug such as gastroenteritis and are being sick all the time, you will still need some insulin to keep your glucose under control. If you can't keep any fluids down, you must call your doctor straightaway. You may have to go into hospital for a while until you are able to eat and drink again.

Type 2

Continuing to take your tablets when you're not able to eat or drink may cause a hypoglycaemic reaction. You may need a lower dose while you're ill but, unless you're monitoring your blood glucose regularly, you may need your doctor's advice on how to make the adjustment. If your illness doesn't settle down quickly, you may be admitted to hospital for a few days.

Having a baby

The fact that you have diabetes is no reason to put off having a baby. The condition does not affect your fertility, and you should have no problems conceiving unless you are one of the minority of women who have severe complications or whose diabetes is poorly controlled.

If you are planning to conceive in the near future, it's a good idea to make sure that your blood glucose levels are as well controlled as possible. In addition, folic acid supplements should be taken.

Babies born to mothers with diabetes are more prone to medical problems with their heart or skeleton, but this risk can be reduced by very careful control of blood glucose levels before pregnancy. Ideally you should talk this over with your diabetes care team – you may find that your hospital offers a special preconceptual counselling service.

You need to watch your blood glucose levels particularly carefully when you're pregnant because, if they get too high, they can affect the baby. This can mean that the baby grows too quickly or too much fluid accumulates in the surrounding membranes.

Your doctor will probably want to see you every few weeks, and you'll also be asked to do your own blood glucose checks more often than usual. It's likely that your insulin dose will double or even treble during this time, but it will go back to normal after the birth. The insulin can't do your baby any harm, because it does not seem to lower the baby's blood glucose, and there's no need to worry that you could injure him or her by injecting into your abdomen. Hypoglycaemia is not known to harm the baby in any way.

There's a good chance that you will be able to have a normal delivery, although some women do have to have a caesarean section. This is because some babies from mothers with diabetes whose glucose levels were higher than ideal may have grown too large for normal vaginal delivery. Your obstetric and diabetes care teams will discuss the options with you beforehand and, if a normal delivery is decided on, you may well have a drip containing insulin and a sugar solution to control your diabetes during labour.

Huge advances in the antenatal care of women with diabetes in recent years mean that, with careful preconceptual preparation and good blood glucose control, you can look forward to a healthy pregnancy and a normal, healthy baby at the end of it.

Pregnancy

You can enjoy a healthy pregnancy and a normal healthy baby at the end of it.

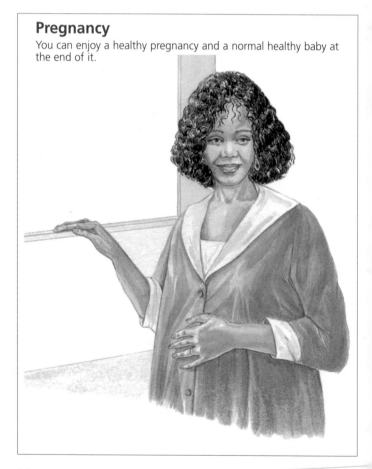

Pregnancy and type 2 diabetes

Type 2 diabetes is becoming more common in younger women who wish to become pregnant. Some tablet treatment is not recommended in pregnancy, so most women need to be switched to insulin, preferably before conception and certainly as soon as possible after pregnancy has been confirmed.

Gestational diabetes

Some women develop diabetes for the first time when they're pregnant, after which their blood glucose levels return to normal. Usually, gestational diabetes, as it's known, can be kept under control by eating the right kinds of foods, although some women do have to have metformin and/or insulin injections.

After the birth, you'll be advised to keep an eye on your weight and stick to a healthy diet because you are at a greater than normal risk of developing type 2 diabetes later in life.

KEY POINTS

■ If planning vigorous exercise, remember to take extra carbohydrate or reduce your insulin or sulphonylurea medication beforehand

■ Remember that vigorous exercise can lead to delayed hypoglycaemia some hours later

■ If exercising with others, always tell them that you have diabetes and explain what to do in the event of a hypoglycaemic attack

■ For parties, remember never to drink alcohol on an empty stomach and have some quick-acting carbohydrate always available

■ If eating later than usual or having extra food, you may need more insulin

■ Remember to take out health insurance before any foreign travel

■ If travelling between continents, when heading west have an extra dose of insulin with your extra meal and when heading east you may omit a scheduled meal and insulin dose

■ Never pack your insulin in your suitcase – keep it in your hand luggage

■ Always carry identification stating your diagnosis and medication

- Even if you are ill and not eating, you still need your insulin

- If you cannot take your medication or insulin because of vomiting, seek medical help

- Diabetic women should try, wherever possible, to plan their pregnancy and seek urgent obstetric and medical advice once they realise that they are pregnant

Children with diabetes

Managing a child's diabetes

Historically, type 1 diabetes most commonly comes on between the ages of 11 and 13. It is, however, becoming more common in toddlers and infants, and there are increasing numbers of cases of babies developing it within a few months of birth.

You can't stop children racing around and burning up energy, which can make it difficult to keep their eating and insulin in the right balance. The usual answer is to give two or three injections a day each containing some short-acting and some medium-acting insulin.

It's only to be expected that you'll worry about your child having hypoglycaemic reactions and find it hard to let him or her out of your sight. As they get older and you both get more used to dealing with diabetes, you'll probably find it easier to allow them more independence.

Children can learn to inject themselves from any age, although you will probably want to check the insulin doses. Injector pens have been a big help in getting around this problem, because of their convenience and ease of dialling the insulin dose.

Children and injecting insulin

Children can learn to inject themselves, but you will probably want to check the insulin doses.

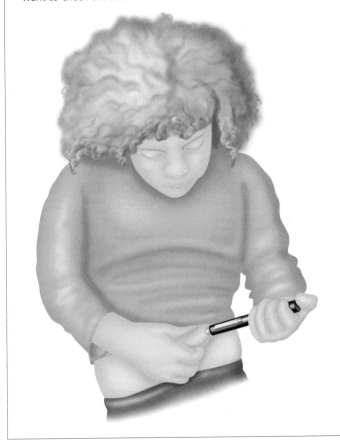

Home monitoring

Blood tests can be hard for young children, and quite difficult because their fingers are so small, so urine tests are sometimes recommended instead, either on their own or combined with occasional blood tests. Once your child is a bit older, you will have to encourage him or her to be disciplined about monitoring blood glucose levels on a regular basis.

However, don't be surprised if he or she is awkward about it. Rebellion is of course a natural part of growing up, and many teenagers go through a period of refusing to cooperate over this aspect of their diabetes care. This is a difficult situation to deal with, but it's best to steer clear of direct confrontation as much as you can. Remember that it's very important for your child to keep taking his or her insulin regularly.

Hypoglycaemia

Children's blood glucose can fall quite quickly, especially if they are active, so it may be difficult to spot the warning signs in time. Very young children may not recognise them at all. When the blood glucose drops so low that the child becomes drowsy or even unconscious, the best treatment is glucagon. It's always worth keeping a supply handy if you are looking after a young child with diabetes.

Once this treatment has worked, the child needs to have some carbohydrate in the form of food or a sweet drink. As the problem is most likely to arise when the child is exercising, it's essential that a playgroup leader, teacher or whoever is in charge (or a friend if the children are unsupervised) knows exactly what to do if he or she does have a hypoglycaemic reaction.

In any case, once your child starts school, it's important that the staff be aware that he or she has diabetes and know what to do in the case of a hypoglycaemic reaction. You will also need to make sure that the kitchen staff are aware of the situation if your child has lunch there, so that he or she makes the appropriate food choices.

Problems with food

The amount that a child eats can vary enormously from one day to the next. If you've ever looked after young children, you'll know how difficult it is to persuade them to eat anything some days, and at other times you can't stop them eating constantly. This obviously makes life rather difficult for you if you have a child with diabetes.

As a rule, your main priority is to give your child something to eat whenever he or she is hungry, even if this means having more than their diet says they should. As children get older, they need bigger doses of insulin, and positive urine tests or high blood glucose values mean that they need more insulin rather than less food.

Low blood glucose, on the other hand, can mean a child needs either less insulin or more food, and this will need to be discussed with his or her diabetes care team.

Many children break the rules and eat sweets or chocolate on the quiet. You shouldn't cut down on their normal food intake to try to compensate for these extra illicit carbohydrates, however. If your child is old enough to understand, try to explain calmly why cheating in this way will result in a high blood glucose, and why this, in turn, may lead to complications (see page 107). Talking the situation over together in a calm and measured way with plenty of time is probably the best approach, although not easy.

Children with diabetes will need to take the same kind of precautions as adults when their normal routine is disrupted, say by travel or illness (see pages 90 and 93). They will also have to learn how to take care of themselves when exercising, and follow the commonsense rules outlined on page 86.

If you are in any doubt about how to handle any of these situations, the team at your child's diabetes clinic will be happy to advise you. The Diabetes UK helpline will also be able to offer advice (see page 147).

Family reactions

When a child with diabetes has brothers or sisters, they may become jealous of the amount of extra attention that he or she gets because of the condition. Equally, children may resent the fact that they have to cope with diabetes when the others don't have to bother.

It's important that all these feelings are brought out into the open and discussed by the whole family. Talking things over – at regular intervals if necessary – can help to clear the air, and may encourage your other children to become involved in watching for signs of hypoglycaemia. If they're old enough and willing, you should teach them how to treat a hypoglycaemic reaction (see page 79).

One area of possible family contention is mealtimes – with complaints from those who don't have diabetes about having to eat healthy foods! The fact is, of course, that the kind of diet recommended for people with diabetes is the same one that we should all be following. It's not much fun for the child who has diabetes if the others constantly eat forbidden treats like sweets and chocolate in front of him or her, so do what you can to discourage this.

Again, talking the situation over and explaining the problem is the approach that's most likely to work and, if you can persuade other children to restrict their sweets intake, it will be good for their health too.

Playing up

Many children quickly discover that being awkward about food is a great way to wind their parents up, and those who have diabetes are no exception. They may well realise that refusing to eat at mealtimes or having a hypoglycaemic reaction is a sure-fire way to get masses of attention. They may also refuse to do urine or blood glucose tests or even make up the results.

This is obviously worrying and frustrating for you as parents, and can cause great disruption to family life. It's not at all unusual, however, and you shouldn't feel guilty because you feel that you can't cope. Your diabetes care team will have seen this kind of problem many times before, and be able to offer help and advice.

Sometimes it can be a good idea to bring in an outsider – a family friend or even a specially trained counsellor – who can help the child concerned to understand the effect that their behaviour is having. It's important to understand that this may sometimes be children's ways of expressing their own deep-seated worries about their diabetes.

KEY POINTS

- Diabetes most commonly comes on between the ages of 11 and 13, although the average age of onset is falling

- Very young children may need to rely on urine tests but older children should be encouraged to use blood tests if possible

- Food battles are even more common and problematic with children with diabetes because of parental anxiety over hypoglycaemia

- Try to avoid confrontation, however, and if battles are causing family upset discuss the issues with your diabetes care team

If it gets complicated

Avoiding complications

The first thing that you need to know is that you will not inevitably develop complications simply because you have diabetes. Careful research has shown that, the better your blood glucose control, the less likely you are to experience any complications.

Large studies in the USA (the Diabetes Control and Complications Trial or DCCT) and the UK (UK Prospective Diabetes Study or UKPDS) have shown that any improvement in blood glucose control will reduce your risk of developing complications.

Knowing this motivates many people to work harder at controlling their diabetes when they're tempted to let things slide a little.

Stop smoking

Along with good diabetic control, giving up (or not starting) smoking can reduce your chances of developing complications. Smoking and diabetes definitely don't mix. All of the possible complications discussed below are more common in people who smoke, and anyone who has already developed any of them should stop smoking immediately. The importance of this can't be overstressed, and knowing that may be the incentive that you need to help you give up if you are a smoker.

Your eyes

Diabetes can affect your eyes in various different ways.

Blurring

When you first start having insulin or tablet treatment, you may notice that your vision seems a bit blurred. This is because the lens in your eye becomes dehydrated when diabetes develops and, by rapidly lowering your blood glucose, the treatment brings about a fluid shift into your eye. This is what causes any blurring.

Fortunately, the problem is only temporary and should clear up in a few months without the need for treatment. If it happens to you, wait until the blurring has disappeared before getting a prescription for new spectacles if you need one. The result of your sight test may well be different once your diabetes has stabilised.

Cataracts

When you have had diabetes for a long time, you are more susceptible to cataracts because of a build-up of sugars in the lens of the eye. These make the lens of your eye opaque, interfering with the transmission of light to the back of your eye, and can be a particular nuisance in bright sunlight.

Fortunately, this problem can be treated quite easily with a simple operation to replace your damaged lens

Places in the body where diabetes can cause complications

The good news is that many of the possible problems can be treated, and often the treatment is most effective when the complications are picked up early. This is why you will be asked to attend regular medical check-ups.

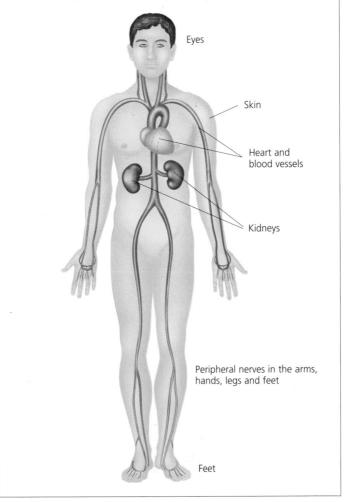

Eyes

Skin

Heart and blood vessels

Kidneys

Peripheral nerves in the arms, hands, legs and feet

Feet

with a plastic one. It can often be done under a local anaesthetic, and you will normally be treated as a day patient. The results are generally excellent.

Retinopathy

Both types of diabetes can affect a highly specialised structure at the back of your eye called the retina. The central part (the macula) enables you to see colours and fine detail, whereas the outer (or peripheral) part picks up black and white and enables you to see in restricted light.

It's the small blood vessels (called capillaries) supplying the retina that are affected by diabetes. This is probably because of a build-up of glucose and other sugars in the walls of the blood vessels, making them weaker.

Small blisters or microaneurysms can form and occasionally burst, resulting in tiny haemorrhages. Sometimes, blood vessels may leak, allowing fluid to collect on the surface of the retina, which then forms what are called hard exudates.

This leakiness is usually a sign that the blood supply to that part of the eye is not as good as it should be. When retinopathy reaches an advanced stage, new blood vessels can grow as the eye tries to improve its blood supply. These new vessels are fragile and may break and bleed extensively. This condition, known as a vitreous haemorrhage, can seriously affect sight.

Treating retinopathy

Fortunately, laser treatment can do a great deal to repair the damage caused by diabetic retinopathy. It's normally directed at the peripheral part of the retina, well away from the macula, and can remove hard

The anatomy of the eye

This illustration shows the principal features of the eye. It is the blood vessels supplying the retina that are mainly affected by diabetes.

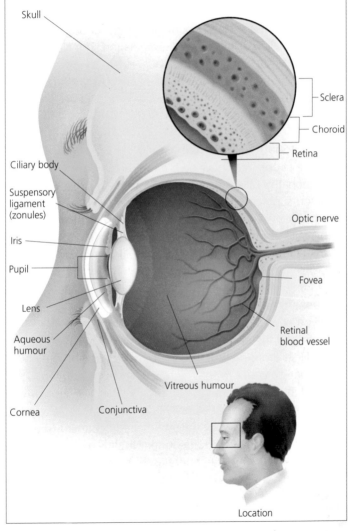

Skull

Sclera

Choroid

Retina

Ciliary body

Suspensory ligament (zonules)

Optic nerve

Iris

Pupil

Fovea

Lens

Aqueous humour

Retinal blood vessel

Cornea

Conjunctiva

Vitreous humour

Location

exudates and prevent new blood vessels from growing. The earlier the treatment is given, the more successful it is, which is why it is essential that you should have your eyes checked at least once a year. ?

Eye checks can be done by an optician or optometrist, a specialist ophthalmologist or a doctor who is skilled at this type of examination. The National Service Framework (NSF) for Diabetes (see page 127) set a deadline for 2007 for an annual photographic eye check to be available for all people with diabetes in England and Wales (earlier for Scotland).

Maculopathy

Some people may develop a more serious form of retinopathy called maculopathy. This means that the blood supply to the central part of the eye is reduced, which can seriously affect the person's ability to perceive colour and fine detail. Unfortunately, laser treatment is not so successful in treating this particular problem.

Laser treatment

If you need laser treatment, you will normally be asked to attend the outpatient clinic at a special eye unit.

First, drops are put into your eye to widen the pupil so that it's easier to see the retina. You then rest your head in a special bracket to keep it still while the doctor uses a type of camera to examine your eye and identify which parts of the retina need treatment (see figure on page 14). The treatment itself is usually painless, but you'll see brief flashes of bright light as the laser is used – sometimes several hundred in each treatment session.

You may need several of these sessions for each eye and, afterwards, your vision could be blurred for about 24 to 48 hours. Extensive laser treatment can reduce the width of vision or visual field and make it harder to see at night. Sometimes the reduction in visual field may have implications for driving.

Vitrectomy

Occasionally for advanced eye disease it is necessary to remove the vitreous humour and replace it with an oil-based liquid. This is called a vitrectomy and is only carried out in specialised vitreoretinal surgery units.

Others

There is intensive research into medical treatment of eye complications. Local injections of steroids into the macula can reduce swelling (oedema). Inhibitors of a growth factor called vascular endothelial growth factor (VEGF) may prevent new vessels from growing. These treatments are, however, still restricted to specialised units.

Your kidneys

One of the main tasks of the kidney is to excrete (get rid of) excess water and the natural chemical byproducts of everyday living via the urine. They do this by filtering the blood through a delicate network of very small vessels called capillaries (similar to those seen at the back of the eye).

As in the eye diabetes can damage these small blood vessels by an accumulation of glucose in the vessel walls. The effect is to allow chemicals and substances that would normally be retained in the

The role of the kidneys

There are usually two kidneys; their function is to excrete urine and to regulate the water, salt composition and acidity of the blood.

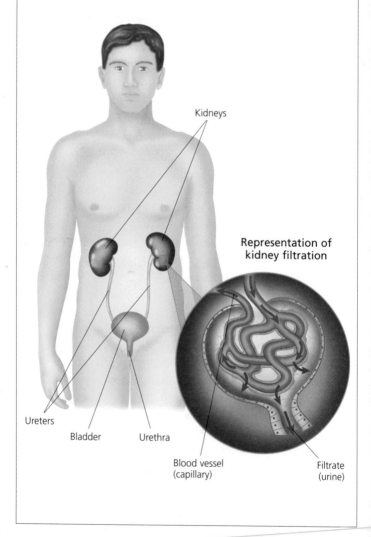

Kidneys

Representation of kidney filtration

Ureters

Bladder

Urethra

Blood vessel
(capillary)

Filtrate
(urine)

blood to pass into the urine. It would be like making holes in a tea strainer larger, which would allow tea leaves to appear in the cup.

One of the substances that appears in the urine when the filters are damaged is protein, and a particular protein called albumin appears at a very early stage of diabetic kidney damage. Albumin in the urine is also called albuminuria and a test can detect the presence of very small amounts (microalbuminuria).

The availability of these tests is one reason why you will probably be asked to provide a urine sample at each of your diabetes clinic visits, even if you are normally performing blood tests for glucose. Sometimes you may get a positive result from the albumin test, which is in fact caused by a urinary infection. Your clinic will check your urine sample to exclude this.

Your doctor will want to keep a closer eye on you if albumin is detected in your urine because there is the possibility of more serious kidney damage and even kidney failure in the long term.

These check-ups are even more important if, like many people with albuminuria, you also have raised blood pressure. The two tend to go together because the kidneys also have a role in controlling blood pressure. Research has shown that careful control of blood pressure in people with diabetes reduces or even prevents kidney damage occurring.

At the moment, those people who developed kidney failure may need treatment either by dialysis (a kidney machine) or by transplantation, but there is a lot of current research into prevention of kidney damage that may one day make this unnecessary.

Your nerves

Diabetes can affect the nerves in two ways: as with the eyes and kidneys, their blood supply may be affected, or there can be direct damage to the nerves themselves as a result of high blood glucose.

Any kind of nerve damage is known medically as neuropathy. The consequences will depend on which of the three types of nerve is affected.

Motor (movement) nerves

These carry messages to the muscles from the brain, stimulating them to contract. Damage to this type of nerve is known as motor neuropathy and can lead to a loss of small muscle activity in the feet or hands. As a result, the toes can become clawed and stick upwards, and the fingers become weak. For more on diabetes and the foot, see page 119.

Sensory nerves

These detect pain, touch, heat and other sensations, and send messages back to the brain. Sensory neuropathy can make the feet very sensitive and even painful at first, but eventually they will become numb and unable to feel any kind of sensation, including pain.

Autonomic nerves

These are responsible for controlling automatic bodily functions such as bowel and bladder activity. Autonomic neuropathy is relatively uncommon, and its most troublesome effects are on the bladder and bowels.

It can result in constipation or diarrhoea that comes and goes, and occasionally the person may suffer from persistent vomiting. Men may also be troubled by a reduction of their sexual potency. Most of these problems can be improved by drug treatment.

Male sexual potency

A man's ability to have a normal erection depends upon a good supply of blood via the arteries leading to the penis, and also on an intact nerve supply. Blood enters the penis through the arteries, which are dilated (made wider) by nerve stimulation as a result of sexual arousal. The extra blood presses on the veins and is therefore trapped in the penis, leading to an erection. Diabetes can affect both the blood supply and the nervous control needed to maintain an erection.

It's important to remember, however, that impotence can have psychological as well as physical causes, whether or not you have diabetes, so it's very important to discuss any sexual problems openly and frankly with your medical advisers.

There are treatments available on prescription for sexual impotence (often called erectile dysfunction or ED) in men with diabetes. Please ask your diabetes care team for advice.

Your skin

A small minority of people with diabetes may have skin problems caused by damage to small blood vessels. When this occurs, it results in reddening and thinning of the skin over the lower shin bones – a condition known as necrobiosis lipoidica. Unfortunately, there is no effective treatment.

Your arteries

Diabetes leads to an increased risk of developing hardening and narrowing of the large blood vessels or

The process of atheroma

Atheroma is the process by which fat is deposited on the inside walls of blood vessels. The deposits can grow to such an extent that they restrict blood flow. They can be treated by angioplasty, stenting or surgical bypass.

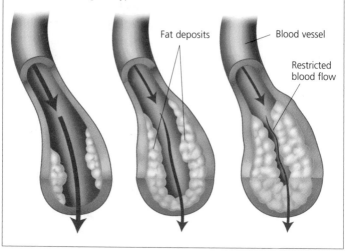

Fat deposits

Blood vessel

Restricted blood flow

arteries, which can lead to heart attacks and strokes, and poor circulation in the legs.

Both smoking and being overweight increase the risk still more, so it is really important that you stop smoking and try to lose weight. In any case, smoking is a known major risk factor for arterial disease even in people who don't have diabetes.

Another factor that can cause arterial disease is a raised blood cholesterol level. Recent research has shown that lowering blood cholesterol with diet and/or medication can lower the risk of heart attacks and strokes.

High blood pressure can also cause hardening of your arteries. Lowering blood pressure has been shown to reduce the risk of heart attacks and strokes, as well as preventing kidney complications (see above).

Problems caused by hardening of the arteries are very common, and there are both medical and surgical treatments available. Narrowed portions of larger arteries can be bypassed by surgical operation, or widened by passing a balloon across them (angioplasty) or using an implanted metal stent. However, it is well worth doing everything that you can to prevent such problems developing in the first place.

Your feet

You need to be aware of changes to your feet that can arise because of your diabetes and what you can do to minimise the risk of damage. Most people with diabetes don't get serious foot problems, but even those who do can prevent things getting worse by caring for their feet properly.

Healthy circulation to your feet will help to keep the tissues strong, and you can encourage this by eating the right kinds of foods, keeping good control of your diabetes and not smoking.

Ensure that your shoes fit well with enough room for your toes, and with a fastening to keep them in place without rubbing. In addition, there are specific things that you can do to look after your feet. These are designed to guard against four changes that can be caused by diabetes.

Poor blood supply to the foot

This results from narrowing of the blood vessels. When your circulation is restricted in this way, your foot is less able to cope with hazards such as cold weather, infection or injury, and is more susceptible to the other three changes

Feet and footwear

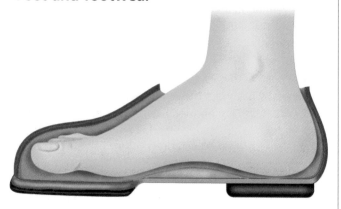

Ensure that your shoes fit correctly – adequate room without being sloppy

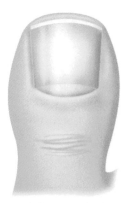

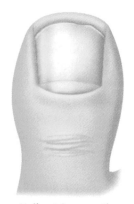

Nail cut correctly
Cut made straight across, not protruding and not trimmed down the sides of the toe

Nail cut incorrectly
Too short and cut down each side

Caring for your feet

Good foot care is very important in preventing complications in diabetes and should form part of your hygiene routine. Feet should be washed and inspected daily.

- Wash your feet daily in warm water using a mild soap. Don't soak them for a long time because it removes more of the precious oils from your skin. You may develop soggy areas between your toes which can split or increase the likelihood of soft corns

- Apply surgical spirit to any white, damp areas between your toes, unless there has been any bleeding. If there has, use dry dressings instead. Any signs of athlete's foot can be treated with surgical spirit, but, if that doesn't work, use an antifungal powder or spray from the chemist

- Your toenails should be cut or filed straight across, unless a state-registered chiropodist (also called a podiatrist) advises otherwise. Sharp corners can be filed over with a foot file or an emery board

- Corns and calluses (hard skin) are best left to the state-registered chiropodist/podiatrist who will either provide or recommend specific protection for the affected areas. Lint pads or cushion soles may be a useful temporary protection for affected areas if you can't get to see the chiropodist/ podiatrist straight away

- Get medical advice immediately if you see any signs of ulceration or infection developing anywhere on your feet

below. Keep your feet warm with good quality socks and stockings, but avoid overheating and be very careful of seams that can press and rub, causing blisters. Consider wearing socks inside out if the seams are prominent.

Neuropathy in the feet

Neuropathy makes the foot less sensitive to pain and temperature. In its early stages, people often complain of pins and needles or a feeling that they are 'walking on cotton wool or pebbles'.

When the ability of your foot to feel is reduced, you're less likely to notice accidental injuries or infection, which will lead to increased damage if nothing is done. In some cases, skin breaks down over a part of the foot that has experienced sustained pressure, because you don't feel the discomfort that would otherwise make you shift your position.

If you are suffering from some degree of neuropathy, you have to get into the habit of checking your feet every day for any cuts or wounds that didn't hurt at the time.

The easiest way is to make a regular foot care programme part of your daily routine. It is also important to check the water temperature with your hand before getting into a bath, and to avoid 'toasting your toes' in front of the fire.

Dryness

Loss of elasticity or dryness in the skin of your feet can be associated with neuropathy and a poor blood supply, but it can develop even when you have good circulation and a normal amount of feeling.

You may notice that your skin is becoming dry even if you haven't had diabetes for very long, and be

Changes that may occur in the foot of a person with diabetes

The following changes are not inevitable and can largely be prevented by good foot hygiene, regular inspection and appropriate care.

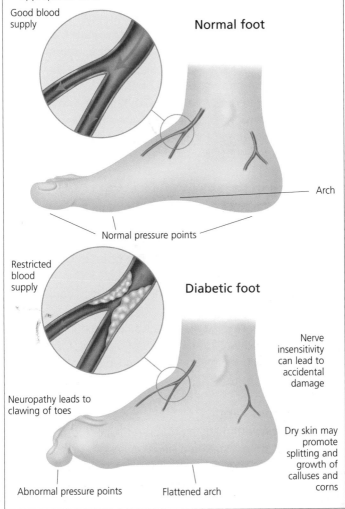

Good blood supply

Normal foot

Arch

Normal pressure points

Restricted blood supply

Diabetic foot

Nerve insensitivity can lead to accidental damage

Neuropathy leads to clawing of toes

Dry skin may promote splitting and growth of calluses and corns

Abnormal pressure points

Flattened arch

inclined to dismiss it as just a minor nuisance. However, dry and flaky skin is much less supple because it is not protected by the sweat and natural oils from the everyday pressures and frictions of walking. When the skin on your feet is very dry, you're more prone to the formation of calluses and corns, and also to splits around the edges (known as fissures).

You can help to replace some of the lost natural moisture by applying a good hand cream every day (to your feet) and using a foot file or pumice stone to remove dead skin. Do be gentle, though, and never, ever use chemicals designed to remove corns and calluses or try to cut them away with blades because you could easily injure yourself.

Changes in the shape of your feet

These can take place over a period of time as a result of neuropathy. The bones underneath may become more prominent as a results of changes in the fatty pad under the ball of your foot. The front part of your foot may spread and your toes may claw. When the tissues under your foot are strained, you may get pain in your heel.

Usually, these changes are a result of minor alterations in the shape of your foot, but don't forget that they could still mean that you need new shoes to get a better fit.

Expert foot care

As a person with diabetes, you are eligible for treatment from a state-registered chiropodist/podiatrist on the NHS – your GP or health centre should have a list of local practitioners. Many people are perfectly able to look after their own feet, but anyone who has a physical or visual disability or any of the complications listed above should have regular appointments with a state-registered chiropodist/podiatrist.

Preventing complications from occurring

You are probably feeling rather alarmed after reading about all these possible complications, so it's worth emphasising again that they can all be prevented by careful attention to diabetes care and blood glucose control.

Remember that complications are not inevitable – and that you have an important role in prevention.

KEY POINTS

- Diabetes can affect the eyes by causing cataracts or damage the back of the eyes – called retinopathy

- Early detection and treatment of eye problems are very effective at preventing progression

- Kidney damage occurs in a minority of patients and can be detected early by a urine test for albumin

- Careful control of blood pressure is an essential part of treatment of diabetes and can protect against kidney complications and hardening of the arteries

- Nerves can also be damaged, and feet and hands need to be checked regularly

- Lowering blood cholesterol by diet and/or medication can reduce the risk of heart attacks and stroke

- Foot care is extremely important in preventing complications

- Feet should be inspected and washed daily, and nails should be cut straight across with sharp edges smoothed off with a file

- Moisturisers can help prevent skin dryness

- Feet should be checked once a year by a health-care professional

Diabetes care

National Service Framework for Diabetes

The Departments of Health in England, Northern Ireland, Wales and Scotland have all produced a National Service Framework (NSF) for Diabetes, which sets out an ambitious list of standards of care to be met by 2013 (earlier in Scotland). There are some differences between each of the countries but the principles are largely the same.

In England, the 12 standards are as set out in the table on page 130 and a summary leaflet entitled *Living with Diabetes: Your future health and well being* (number 29335) is available from the Department of Health (see page 146 for the address).

There were two clear milestones in the English NSF:

1 All people with diabetes were to have access to annual eye photography for screening for retinopathy by 2007.
2 All GP surgeries were to have an up-to-date register and systematic programme of care for people with diabetes by 2006.

Whereas universal eye screening is available in most parts of the UK, the second milestone has yet to be universally achieved.

The new contract for GPs specifies certain important targets for all of their patients with diabetes. This means that there are strong incentives to provide comprehensive care at your local surgery.

Contact your health centre or surgery for details of what care is available. It is also proposed to set up locally managed care networks made up of health-care professionals, people with diabetes and their carers, to make sure that there is progress towards meeting all the standards by 2013.

This process is to be supervised by the National Clinical Director for Diabetes. The NSF actively encourages involvement in this process and a local lay champion is to be appointed in every district.

To find out more about how you can get involved you can contact your local primary care trust, NHS Direct (see page 150), Diabetes UK (see page 147) or the Department of Health website (see page 146).

What care should you expect?

Medical and lay members of Diabetes UK have drawn up a charter (see below) of what you should expect from your medical carers.

Newly diagnosed

When you have just been diagnosed, you should have:

- A full medical examination.

- A talk with a registered nurse who has a special interest in diabetes. She or he will explain what diabetes is and talk to you about your individual treatment.

- A talk with a state-registered dietitian, who will want to know what you are used to eating and will give you basic advice on what to eat in the future. A follow-up meeting should be arranged for more detailed advice.

- A discussion of the implications of your diabetes for your job, driving, insurance, prescription charges, etc. and whether you need to inform the DVLA and your insurance company, if you are a driver.

- Information about Diabetes UK's services and details of your local Diabetes UK group.

- Ongoing education about your diabetes and the beneficial effects of exercise, and assessments of your control.

You should be able to take a close friend or relative with you to educational sessions if you wish.

Insulin treatment

If you are treated with insulin, you should have:

- Frequent sessions for basic instruction on injection technique, looking after insulin and syringes and pens, blood glucose testing and what the results mean.

- Supplies of relevant equipment.

- Discussion about hypoglycaemia (a hypo) and how to deal with it.

NSF Standards for Diabetes Care

Standard 1: Prevention

The NHS will reduce the overall risk of people developing diabetes.

Standard 2: Identifying/Screening for Diabetes

The NHS will develop programmes for screening for type 2 diabetes.

Standard 3: Patient Empowerment

The NHS will give people with diabetes the information to enable them to take part in decisions about their care. Newly diagnosed people with diabetes will be assigned a named health-care professional who will help them learn how to look after their diabetes.

Standard 4: Clinical Care – Adults

All adults will receive high-quality care including information and support to reduce the risk of developing diabetes complications.

Standards 5 and 6: Clinical Care – Children and Young People

All children and young people will receive equally high-quality care, which will be extended to their carers. Clinical services will be developed to enable a smooth transfer of children from paediatric to adult services.

Standard 7 Clinical Care – Diabetic Emergencies

Diabetes services will have in place evidence-based

in England – to be achieved by 2013

protocols for quick and effective treatment of diabetic emergencies including comas.

Standard 8: Clinical Care – Diabetes Patients in Hospital

All people with diabetes who are in hospital will receive informed and effective care of their condition whatever their reason for being an inpatient.

Standard 9: Clinical Care – Pregnancy

All women with diabetes wishing to become pregnant or who are pregnant or develop diabetes during their pregnancy will receive high-quality care to protect their health and to maximise the chance of a normal healthy baby.

Standard 10: Identifying and Treating Complications

All people with diabetes will receive regular checks to identify long-term complications.

Standards 11 and 12: Treating Complications and Providing Support

Long-term complications will be identified and treated at an early stage in order to reduce the risk of permanent disability or early death. The NHS will also work closely with all other relevant organisations in order to provide joint care for people with diabetes.

Full details of standards available from the Department of Health website (see 'Useful addresses', page 146).

Tablet treatment

If you are treated by tablets, you should have:

- A discussion about the possibility of hypoglycaemia (a hypo) and how to deal with it.

- Instruction on blood or urine testing and what the results mean and supplies of relevant equipment.

Dietary treatment alone

If you are treated by diet alone, you should have instruction on blood or urine testing and what the results mean and supplies of relevant equipment.

Ongoing care

Once your diabetes is reasonably controlled, you should:

- Have access to the diabetes team at regular intervals – annually if necessary. These meetings should give time for discussion as well as assessing diabetes control.

- Be able to contact any member of the health-care team for specialist advice when you need it.

- Have more education sessions as you are ready for them.

- Have a formal medical review once a year by a doctor experienced in diabetes.

At this review:

- Your weight should be recorded.
- Your urine should be tested for protein.
- Your blood should be tested to measure long-term control.

- You should discuss control, including your home monitoring results.

- Your blood pressure should be checked.

- Your vision should be checked and the back of your eyes examined. A photograph may be taken of the back of your eyes. If necessary, you should be referred to an ophthalmologist.

- Your legs and feet should be examined to check your circulation and nerve supply. If necessary, you should be referred to a state-registered chiropodist/podiatrist.

- If you are on insulin, your injection sites should be examined.

- You should have the opportunity to discuss how you are coping at home and at work.

The importance of your involvement

You are an important member of the care team, so it is essential that you understand your own diabetes to enable you to be in control of your own condition.

You should ensure that you receive the described care from your local diabetes clinic, practice or hospital. If these services are not available, you should:

- Contact your GP to discuss the diabetes care available in your area

- Contact your local primary care trust

- Contact Diabetes UK or your local branch (see page 147).

Future prospects for people with diabetes

Advances in prevention, cure and treatment

As diabetes is a common condition and seems to be increasing in incidence worldwide, there is a great deal of research into prevention, cures and treatment of any complications.

Prevention

The ideal treatment would be to prevent diabetes occurring at all. Our understanding of the causes of diabetes has increased dramatically over the last few decades but there is still much to be learnt.

In particular we do not understand what it is that triggers the damage to the small beta (β) cells that produce insulin in the pancreas. The genes that predispose patients to this damage are being identified but precisely what they control and how the damage is initiated remain unclear.

Nevertheless, once these questions are answered it is perhaps feasible that repairing these genes in patients at risk of diabetes could prevent them developing the condition, although such developments are a long way from being a practical option.

Two studies from Finland and the USA have shown that modest exercise of around three hours' brisk walking per week, combined with a weight loss of around five per cent, can dramatically reduce the risk of people with impaired glucose tolerance going on to develop type 2 diabetes.

These results emphasise the importance of healthy living, exercise and weight control as the best way of preventing type 2 diabetes.

Recent research in the UK has raised the exciting prospect of a vaccine to prevent type 1 diabetes. This preliminary work is unlikely to lead to widespread treatment for some time, however.

Cures and treatments

Many patients ask if it is possible to have a transplant to cure their diabetes. For patients with type 1 diabetes this is an attractive prospect. If it were possible to isolate the small beta cells that make insulin and then either inject them or replace them in the patient, insulin production should be restored.

There has been a great deal of research in this area over the last few decades, but a major problem remains with rejection of the transplanted cells. In addition, actually collecting the cells from the pancreas of donors is extremely laborious and time-consuming, and there would never be enough of these cells to supply all the people with diabetes worldwide.

Recently, however, scientists in Canada have developed a new technique for both extracting and transplanting islet cells. They have used a powerful combination of anti-rejection drugs, which avoid steroids, and as a result some patients have remained free from insulin injections for several years.

These promising results have led to a large research study being funded by Diabetes UK to see if they can be reproduced over here. In 2005 the first successful transplant using this technique was reported in the UK. This treatment has recently been approved by NICE.

New approaches taking cells from other animals or small segments of the skin of patients with diabetes, and transforming them into insulin-producing cells, are eliciting a great deal of interest.

There is also research into converting stem cells (cells in the body that retain the ability to be changed into any other specialised cell) into insulin-producing cells.

Finally, scientists have recently been able to reprogram liver cells in mice to make insulin by using genetic engineering. Many problems remain with these ideas, although it is possible that trials may start within the next five to ten years.

For people with type 2 diabetes, the problem is more complicated because they may be making insulin but are resistant to its action. New tablets such as the thiazolidinediones (glitazones) improve insulin sensitivity and it is very likely that newer medicines that improve this will be developed in the not too distant future. New compounds that are showing particular promise are islet amyloid polypeptide, which is a naturally occurring substance that lowers blood glucose, and the newer agents that act on GLP-1 (see page 49).

Insulin itself has been chemically altered to change the rate at which it is absorbed from under the skin. This has led to the development of quicker-acting and longer-acting types and some of these new 'analogues' are already available on prescription. This will provide greater flexibility for patients, particularly those with more irregular mealtimes. There is intense research into developing insulin that it will be possible to take by mouth.

Treatments to reduce the complications of diabetes

For the vast majority of patients it is important to discover new treatments to prevent or reduce the risk of developing some of the more serious complications.

These treatments will concentrate on some of the basic mechanisms that cause eye, kidney and nerve damage. As mentioned in 'If it gets complicated' (page 107), it seems that the exposure of these delicate structures to high glucose values for a prolonged period of time causes chemical changes, leading to retinopathy, nephropathy and neuropathy.

Chemicals have been developed to interfere in this process in subtle ways and it may be that long-term treatment with these medicines will prevent complications. Clinical trials are both ongoing and in the early stages of planning.

Careful control of blood pressure and cholesterol levels has also been shown to be effective and it is likely that newer treatments in these areas will be developed in the next few years.

It is important to remember, however, that much can be done to reduce the risks of problems from your diabetes by regular care by both yourself and your diabetes care team. Structured supervision and examination of your eyes, urine tests, blood pressure, feet and tests for cholesterol can indicate areas for treatment that can prevent complications. Already the range of treatments and understanding of the disease have greatly improved the outlook for patients with diabetes and I am sure that this progress will be continued in the future.

KEY POINTS

- Prevention of diabetes remains distant for type 1 diabetes, but careful diet, regular exercise and weight control reduce the chances of developing type 2 diabetes

- Cure of insulin deficiency by transplanting or modifying cells to make insulin is the subject of intensive research

- New treatments to prevent or reverse complications are currently being developed and tested

Questions and answers

Some questions come up time and again when people find out that they have diabetes – here are the answers to some of the most common ones.

- **Will I lose my driving licence because I have diabetes?**

The short answer to this question is no. However, you do have to let the DVLA (Driver and Vehicle Licensing Agency, see page 147), at Swansea know when your diabetes is first diagnosed, unless your treatment consists of diet alone. You'll find the address on your licence. The DVLA will issue you with a three-year licence; then, on the anniversary of renewal, you'll get a questionnaire from them to fill in. Depending on circumstances, you may be asked to see your GP or local diabetes clinic for a brief medical examination before your licence is renewed. You must be fully aware of hypoglycaemia and meet all required visual standards. Patients who have had extensive laser treatment should check at their eye clinic if they meet the requirements.

From January 1998, a European Community Directive on driving regulations came into effect. Motor vehicles are divided into four categories: categories A and B include motorcycles and motor vehicles under 3.5 tonnes in weight. These categories are not affected by the new regulations for patients with diabetes.

However, categories C (motor vehicles over 3.5 tonnes but under 7.5 tonnes) and D (motor vehicles used for carrying passengers with more than eight but fewer than sixteen seats) will require a medical questionnaire to be completed. This has the same standards as the current LGV (large goods vehicle) and PCV (passenger-carrying vehicle) licences and patients needing insulin will normally be excluded from driving vehicles in these classes, unless they were on injections before the rules came into effect.

Diabetes UK has been able to negotiate a concession for category C licence applications for people on insulin. There is an application pack available from the DVLA. A medical examination is required and you would be expected to pay for this (possibly up to £94). If you satisfy the requirements they will send you a further medical questionnaire and you will need a second medical examination from a specialist, which may cost up to a further £100.

If a licence is awarded you will need annual assessments but should not incur any costs for these. Unfortunately no concession has been granted for category D except on a voluntary basis. You can drive a vehicle that weighs less than 3.5 tonnes and has no more than 16 seats, provided that it is strictly on a 'not for hire or reward basis', you are aged between 21 and 70 years, and you have had a category B licence for at least 2 years. The law does not bar insulin users from driving taxis with fewer than nine seats, but many local taxi-licensing authorities do impose restrictions.

As well as the DVLA, you need to let your motor insurance company know if your diabetes develops while the policy is in force. Some companies tend to load premiums for drivers with diabetes and, if this happens to you, contact Diabetes UK (address on page 147) for their list of insurers offering preferential rates for drivers with the condition.

The DVLA has just issued advice for drivers on insulin. They require them to test before driving and at least every two hours if on a long trip. They advise that you should not drive if your glucose is below 4 mmol/l ('four is the floor'). If it is between 4.1 and 5.0 mmol/l they suggest a carbohydrate snack or meal before setting off. If you experience hypoglycaemia when driving, you should pull over, switch off the engine and leave the vehicle, as well as take carbohydrate to raise blood glucose levels.

● **Can I still enjoy a normal sex life?**
Unless a man with diabetes has impotence problems (see page 117), there is no reason why your sex life should be affected in any way and having diabetes makes no difference to a woman's fertility (see page 94). It's worth pointing out, however, that sexual intercourse is a vigorous activity and so could cause your blood glucose level to drop and precipitate a hypoglycaemic reaction in people on insulin, sulphonylureas or glitinides.

● **Can diabetes affect my job?**
It depends to some extent on what you do. The main factor to consider, if you are on insulin or

sulphonylureas, is what the consequences would be for both yourself and your colleagues if you suffered a hypoglycaemic reaction. For this reason, you would have to think carefully about whether to take up a job that involves physical hazards – such as working at heights like a steeplejack or scaffolder – or other dangers, in the police or ambulance services, for example. However, if you were already employed in one of these areas when your condition was first diagnosed, you may be able to carry on if your diabetes is well controlled and you rarely experience hypoglycaemic reactions.

Whatever you do, it is important to tell your employer and your colleagues that you have diabetes, however tempting it might be to keep quiet. It could be very embarrassing and possibly dangerous for you and everyone else if you were to have a hypoglycaemic reaction and no one recognised it or knew what to do.

If you experience difficulties with your job or feel that you might be experiencing discrimination, please contact Diabetes UK for advice. They may be able to put you in contact with individuals or groups who can help. There are new guidelines recently published from professional bodies representing the police and fire services and these are available from Diabetes UK.

• Will my children get diabetes?

For patients with type 1 (insulin-dependent) diabetes, there is a small but increased risk of their children also being affected. For unknown reasons, this is more likely if the father has diabetes. If both parents have diabetes the risk is increased further. At present estimates the risk for a child with one parent with diabetes is around 5 per cent and if both parents have the condition it may be as high as 15 per cent.

For type 2 diabetes (non-insulin dependent), the situation is much less clear. Some families with special types of diabetes have a very high risk of inheritance. These are, however, a very small minority and, for most patients with type 2 diabetes, the risk cannot be determined with any accuracy.

- **Will I go blind or have kidney failure with diabetes?**

As there is a tendency for diabetes to run in families, many patients have direct experience of relatives or acquaintances who have had severe complications from diabetes. As far as eye and kidney problems are concerned, these affect only a minority of patients and the risks of developing problems can be greatly reduced with careful control of blood glucose.

There are also many new treatments available for both eye and kidney complications that can prevent progression or deterioration, provided that the problem is picked up at an early stage. This is why it is critical that patients with diabetes receive regular check-ups.

Useful addresses

We have included the following organisations because, on preliminary investigation, they may be of use to the reader. However, we do not have first-hand experience of each organisation and so cannot guarantee the organisation's integrity. The reader must therefore exercise his or her own discretion and judgement when making further enquiries.

Age UK
York House, 207–221 Pentonville Road
London N1 9UZ
Tel: 0800 169 8787 (8.30am–5pm).
Website: www.ageuk.org

Lots of useful advice, information and fact sheets. Has contact addresses in Scotland, Wales and Northern Ireland.

Association of Blind and Partially Sighted Teachers and Students (ABAPSTAS)
BM Box 6727

London WC1N 3XX
Tel: 01484 690521
Website: www.abapstas.org.uk

Originally supporting visually impaired students, teachers and lecturers, now a national self-help and campaigning organisation with main focus on education and employment. Organises days on study skills, teaching techniques and confidence building.

Benefits Enquiry Line
Tel: 0800 882200
Minicom: 0800 243355
Website: www.dwp.gov.uk
N. Ireland: 0800 220674

Government agency giving information and advice on sickness and disability benefits for people with disabilities and their carers.

Blood Pressure Association
60 Cranmer Terrace
London SW17 0QS
Tel: 020 8772 4994
Information line: 0845 241 0989 (Mon–Fri 11am–3pm)
Website: www.bpassoc.org.uk

Raises public awareness about, and offers information and support to health-care professionals and people affected by high blood pressure. Has a wide selection of literature and membership scheme. A4 envelope and two first-class stamps requested.

Carers UK
20 Great Dover Street
London SE1 4LX
Tel: 020 7378 4999
Carers' line: 0808 808 7777 (Wed, Thurs 10am–12
noon, 2–4pm)
Website: www.carersuk.org

Offers information and support to all people who are
unpaid carers, looking after others with medical or
other problems.

Clinical Knowledge Summaries
Sowerby Centre for Health Informatics at Newcastle
(SCHIN Ltd)
Bede House, All Saints Business Centre
Newcastle upon Tyne NE1 2ES
Tel: 0191 243 6100
Website: www.cks.library.nhs.uk

A website mainly for GPs giving information for patients
listed by disease plus named self-help organisations.

Department of Health (DH)
Richmond House
79 Whitehall, London SW1A 2NS
Website: www.doh.gov.uk

Produces and distributes literature about general health
matters including *Health Advice for Travellers*, also
available on their website. Can apply online for
European Health Insurance Cards (EHICs) for use when
travelling to the EU.

Diabetes UK
Macleod House, 10 Parkway
London NW1 7AA
Tel: 020 7424 1000
Supporter services: 0845 123 2399 (Mon–Fri, 9am–5pm)
Website: www.diabetes.org.uk

Provides valuable advice and information, including
translation service, for people with diabetes, whether
members or not, and their families. Has local support
groups; runs holidays for children and weekends for
families. Members receive magazine *Balance*, free, six
times a year.

Disabled Living Foundation
380–384 Harrow Road
London W9 2HU
Tel: 020 7289 6111
Helpline: 0845 130 9177 (Mon–Fri 10am–4pm)
Website: www.dlf.org.uk

Provides information to disabled and elderly people on
all kinds of equipment in order to promote their
independence and quality of life.

DVLA (Driver and Vehicle Licensing Agency)
DVLA
Swansea SA6 7JL
Tel: 0870 600 0301 (Mon–Fri 8am–5.30pm, Sat 8am–1pm)
Website: www.dvla.gov.uk

Provides advice and information leaflets about diabetes
and driving.

Food Standards Agency
Aviation House, 125 Kingsway
London WC2B 6NH
Helpline: 020 7276 8829
Website: www.food.gov.uk

Advice on diet and health. Wide-ranging information
on additives, contaminants and chemical safety.

INPUT
Tel: 0800 228 9977
Website: www.input.me.uk

Patient-led support group for people using insulin
pumps to control their diabetes.

Insulin Dependent Diabetes Trust
PO Box 294
Northampton NN1 4XS
Tel: 01604 622837
Website: www.iddtinternational.org

Charity supporting and campaigning on behalf of people
with diabetes who experience problems when switching
from one type of insulin to another; in particular
champions the retention of animal insulin for those who
may be intolerant of other, newer forms of insulin.

MedicAlert Foundation
1 Bridge Wharf, 156 Caledonian Road
London N1 9UU
Tel: 0800 581420
Website: www.medicalert.org.uk

A life-saving body-worn identification system for people with hidden medical conditions. The 24-hour emergency telephone number accepts reverse charge calls; can access personal details from anywhere in the world in over 100 languages. Offers selection of jewellery with internationally recognised medical symbol.

mobilise
(Promoting mobility for disabled people)
National Headquarters, Ashwellthorpe
Norwich NR16 1EX
Tel: 01508 489449
Website: www.mobilise.info

Self-help association offering information and advice, and campaigning for independence through mobility with a wide range of services.

National Institute for Health and Clinical Excellence (NICE)
MidCity Place, 71 High Holborn
London WC1V 6NA
Tel: 0845 003 7780
Website: www.nice.org.uk

Provides national guidance on the promotion of good health and treatment of ill-health. Patient information leaflets are available for each piece of guidance issued.

NHS Direct
Tel: 0845 4647 (24 hours, 365 days a year)
Website: www.nhsdirect.nhs.uk

Offers confidential health-care advice, information and referral service. A good first port of call for any health advice.

NHS Smoking Helpline
Freephone: 0800 022 4332 (7am–11pm, 365 days a year)
Website: http://smokefree.nhs.uk
Pregnancy smoking helpline: 0800 169 9169
(12 noon–9pm, 365 days a year)

Have advice, help and encouragement on giving up smoking. Specialist advisers available to offer ongoing support to those who genuinely are trying to give up smoking. Can refer to local branches.

Patients' Association
PO Box 935
Harrow, Middlesex HA1 3YJ
Helpline: 0845 608 4455
Tel: 020 8423 9111
Website: www.patients-association.com

Provides advice on patients' rights, leaflets and a directory of self-help groups.

Quit (Smoking Quitlines)
63 St Mary's Axe
London EC3 8AA
Helpline: 0800 002200 (9am–9pm, 365 days a year)
Tel: 020 7469 0400
Website: www.quit.org.uk

Offers individual advice on giving up smoking in English and Asian languages. Talks to schools on smoking and pregnancy and can refer to local support groups. Runs training courses for professionals.

Royal National Institute of Blind People (RNIB)
105 Judd Street
London WC1H 9NE
Tel: 020 7388 1266
Helpline: 0303 123 9999 (Mon–Fri 8.45am–6pm, Sat 9am–4pm)
Website: www.rnib.org.uk

Offers a range of information and advice on lifestyle changes and employment for people facing loss of sight. Also offers support and training in Braille. Has mail order catalogue of useful aids.

Weight Watchers
Millennium House, Ludlow Road
Maidenhead SL6 2SL
Website: www.weightwatchers.co.uk

Runs informal, yet structured, weekly meetings across the UK for people wanting to lose weight and learn more about living a healthy lifestyle. Guidance also available free with online programme.

Useful websites
BBC
www.bbc.co.uk/health
A helpful website: easy to navigate and offers lots of useful advice and information. Also contains links to other related topics.

Bodytalkonline
www.bodytalk-online.com
Series of online presentations about different medical conditions.

Healthtalkonline
www.healthtalkonline.org
Website of the DIPEx charity.

Patient UK
www.patient.co.uk
Patient care website.

The internet as a source of further information

After reading this book, you may feel that you would like further information on the subject. The internet is of course an excellent place to look and there are many websites with useful information about medical disorders, related charities and support groups.

For those who do not have a computer at home some bars and cafes offer facilities for accessing the internet. These are listed in the *Yellow Pages* under 'Internet Bars and Cafes' and 'Internet Providers'. Your local library offers a similar facility and has staff to help you find the information that you need.

It should always be remembered, however, that the internet is unregulated and anyone is free to set up a website and add information to it. Many websites offer impartial advice and information that have been compiled and checked by qualified medical professionals. Some, on the other hand, are run by commercial organisations with the purpose of promoting their own products. Others still are run by pressure groups, some of which will provide carefully assessed and accurate information whereas others may be suggesting medications or treatments that are not supported by the medical and scientific community.

Unless you know the address of the website you want to visit – for example, www.familydoctor.co.uk – you may find the following guidelines useful when searching the internet for information.

Search engines and other searchable sites

Google (www.google.co.uk) is the most popular search engine used in the UK, followed by Yahoo! (http://uk.yahoo.com) and MSN (www.msn.co.uk). Also popular are the search engines provided by Internet Service Providers such as Tiscali and other sites such as the BBC site (www.bbc.co.uk).

In addition to the search engines that index the whole web, there are also medical sites with search facilities, which act almost like mini-search engines, but cover only medical topics or even a particular area of medicine. Again, it is wise to look at who is responsible for compiling the information offered to ensure that it is impartial and medically accurate. The NHS Direct site (www.nhsdirect.nhs.uk) is an example of a searchable medical site.

Links to many British medical charities can be found at the Association of Medical Research Charities' website (www.amrc.org.uk) and at Charity Choice (www.charitychoice.co.uk).

Search phrases

Be specific when entering a search phrase. Searching for information on 'cancer' will return results for many different types of cancer as well as on cancer in general. You may even find sites offering astrological information. More useful results will be returned by using search phrases such as 'lung cancer' and 'treatments for lung cancer'. Both Google and Yahoo! offer an advanced search option that includes the ability to search for the exact phrase; enclosing the search phrase in quotes, that is, 'treatments for lung cancer', will have the same effect. Limiting a search to an exact phrase reduces the number of results returned but it is best to refine a search to an exact match only if you are not getting useful results with a normal search. Adding 'UK' to your search term will bring up mainly British sites, so a good phrase might be 'lung cancer' UK (don't include UK within the quotes).

Always remember that the internet is international and unregulated. It holds a wealth of valuable information but individual sites may be biased, out of date or just plain wrong. Family Doctor Publications accepts no responsibility for the content of links published in this series.

Index

Your pages

We have included the following pages because they may help you manage your illness or condition and its treatment.

Before an appointment with a health professional, it can be useful to write down a short list of questions of things that you do not understand, so that you can make sure that you do not forget anything.

Some of the sections may not be relevant to your circumstances.

We are always pleased to receive constructive criticism or suggestions about how to improve the books. You can contact us at:

Email: familydoctor@btinternet.com
Letter: Family Doctor Publications
PO Box 4664
Poole
BH15 1NN

Thank you

Health-care contact details

Name:

Job title:

Place of work:

Tel:

Name:

Job title:

Place of work:

Tel:

Name:

Job title:

Place of work:

Tel:

Name:

Job title:

Place of work:

Tel:

Significant past health events – illnesses/operations/investigations/treatments

Event	Month	Year	Age (at time)

Appointments for health care

Name:

Place:

Date:

Time:

Tel:

Name:

Place:

Date:

Time:

Tel:

Name:

Place:

Date:

Time:

Tel:

Name:

Place:

Date:

Time:

Tel:

Appointments for health care

Name:

Place:

Date:

Time:

Tel:

Name:

Place:

Date:

Time:

Tel:

Name:

Place:

Date:

Time:

Tel:

Name:

Place:

Date:

Time:

Tel:

Current medication(s) prescribed by your doctor

Medicine name:

Purpose:

Frequency & dose:

Start date:

End date:

Medicine name:

Purpose:

Frequency & dose:

Start date:

End date:

Medicine name:

Purpose:

Frequency & dose:

Start date:

End date:

Medicine name:

Purpose:

Frequency & dose:

Start date:

End date:

Other medicines/supplements you are taking, not prescribed by your doctor

Medicine/treatment:

Purpose:

Frequency & dose:

Start date:

End date:

Medicine/treatment:

Purpose:

Frequency & dose:

Start date:

End date:

Medicine/treatment:

Purpose:

Frequency & dose:

Start date:

End date:

Medicine/treatment:

Purpose:

Frequency & dose:

Start date:

End date:

Questions to ask at appointments
(Note: do bear in mind that doctors work under great time pressure, so long lists may not be helpful for either of you)

Questions to ask at appointments
(Note: do bear in mind that doctors work under great time
pressure, so long lists may not be helpful for either of you)

Notes

Notes

Notes